The Environmental Pendulum

The Environmental Pendulum

*A Quest for the Truth About Toxic
Chemicals, Human Health, and
Environmental Protection*

R. Allan Freeze

UNIVERSITY OF CALIFORNIA PRESS
Berkeley   Los Angeles   London

University of California Press
Berkeley and Los Angeles, California

University of California Press, Ltd.
London, England

© 2000 by R. Allan Freeze

Library of Congress Cataloging-in-Publication Data

Freeze, R. Allan.
    The environmental pendulum : a quest for the truth about toxic
chemicals, human health, and environmental protection /
R. Allan Freeze.
        p.   cm.
    Includes bibliographical references and index.
    ISBN 0-520-22046-3 (alk. paper).—ISBN 0-520-22047-1 (pbk. : alk.
paper)
    1. Hazardous wastes—Environmental aspects.   2. Hazardous wastes—
Health aspects.   3. Hazardous waste site remediation.   I. Title.
TD1050.E58F74   2000
363.738'4—dc21   99-11340
                                                                      CIP

Manufactured in the United States of America

08   07   06   05   04   03   02   01   00   99
10   9   8   7   6   5   4   3   2   1

The paper used in this publication is both acid-free and totally chlorine-
free (TCF). It meets the minimum requirements of ANSI/NISO Z39.48-1992
(R 1997) (*Permanence of Paper*).

To the next generation: Brenna, Danielle, and Danica

Contents

Illustrations

Tables

Acknowledgments

I have benefited from many discussions, both scientific and philosophical, over many years with many colleagues. At the risk of offending others, let me single out John Cherry, Dave McWhorter, Stavros Papadopulos, Tom Maddock, John Bredehoeft, Pat Domenico, Ghislain de Marsily, Steve Gorelick, Frank Schwartz, Nick Johnson, Paul Witherspoon, Stan Feenstra, and Myles Parsons.

The University of British Columbia was my academic home for many years. In the final few years, I worked with a gifted group of colleagues and students on a set of research topics purposely designed to straddle the boundary between the technical and social aspects of environmental decision-making. I learned much from my interactions with Leslie Smith, Joel Massmann, Tony Sperling, Bruce James, and Dan Walker.

I am very appreciative of the encouragement and critical reading that I received from many friends and colleagues on various parts of the book. In particular, thanks go to John Cherry, Tony Hodge, Tom and Meg Brown, Geoff Freeze, and Rick Freeze. Any errors that remain are mine.

The figures were drafted by Gord Hodge with his usual skill.

Much of this book was written during a delightful sojourn at the Polytechnic University in Valencia, Spain, with the encouragement and support of my colleagues there, Jaime Gomez-Hernandez and Andres Sahuquillo.

I also want to thank those who got me involved in many of the sites highlighted in the book, and who educated me in their technical issues and social complexities: Charlie Andrews, Gerry Grizak, Richard Szudy, Fred Wolf, Tom Sale, Terry Foreman, Beth Parker, Gary Costanzo, Dick Jackson, Ted O'Neill, Rolf Bernegger, Mike Brother, Sybil Hatch, Dave Ketcheson, Paul Kaplan, Dave Donohue, Bob Mutch, and Dale Stephenson.

Finally, I appreciate the efforts of my agent, Sheree Bykofsky, on my behalf, and the support and editing skills of Howard Boyer, Jean McAneny, and Bonita Hurd at the University of California Press.

Prologue

A DAY AT SMITHVILLE

The wind whistled across the grassy field. It was neatly mowed and could have passed for a practice field for the local high school football team. There were about eight of us standing at one end, our tailored suits flapping in the wind, ill-fitting hard hats perched on our heads. We looked like a clutch of ivy league politicians on a blue-collar field trip.

Ted O'Neill was directing our attention to the far end of the field, about where the far goal line would have been if this really were a football field. Instead of goalposts, there were eight little sheds in view. Even at this distance we could hear the whirr of the pumps inside two or three of them.

"Don't be confused by the parklike setting," Ted cautioned us. "They cleaned up the mess on the surface back in the seventies. The real mess is still here, right beneath our feet."

Ted paused as we all looked down at our feet. "The center of the contaminated plume is just over there," he explained, "about twenty feet below the ground surface. There's contamination in the soil, and in the fractured rock that lies below the soil, and in the groundwater that flows through the rock. We've got oils, and solvents, and of course, the PCBs." We all knew about the PCBs because that was why we were there.

"The PCBs don't move far," he said. "They tend to glom onto the rock." He pointed toward the pump sheds. "At most, they might have migrated out as far as the pumps."

"But not beyond?" someone asked.

"We don't think so," Ted answered. "You can see our monitoring wells a little past the pumps. They're clean." He thought for a moment. "Well, not totally clean, of course. We have solvents out there. TCE, PCE, a few others. But no PCBs."

He went on. "Mind you, just because we don't see them in the monitoring wells isn't proof positive that they aren't out there. We don't have x-ray vision. But we think we have containment. We don't think the PCBs are moving past the pumps."

Smithville is a small town in southern Ontario, a few hours' drive from Toronto. In the late seventies, the Smithville site was set up as a hazardous waste transfer station. Barrels of liquid waste and rows of used electrical transformers were stacked up in the back forty like used Chevys in a junkyard. The barrels and transformers were full of PCB oils. Many of them leaked. The fluids seeped down through the surficial soils into the underlying bedrock. Nobody really thought much about it.

Now, in 1996, people were thinking a lot about it. Studies of the site indicated that the groundwater was heavily contaminated. The town wells had been shut down as a health precaution. At a deeper level, the citizens of Smithville felt violated. The town sits in one of the most fertile and pristine rural areas of southern Ontario. The area is known for its heritage homes, its craft shops, its orchards, fruit stalls, and cottage wineries. It does not want to be known as the home of one of North America's most contaminated sites.

The original owners of the transformer station are long gone, lost in the corporate mists of mergers and buyouts and bankruptcies. In Canada such contaminated sites are known as "orphan sites," and like real-life orphans, they usually end up in government care. Some years earlier, the government of Ontario had established the Smithville Bedrock Remediation Program. By 1996 the program was already into Phase IV, and not much had really happened. Ted O'Neill had been brought in to make things happen.

John Cherry and I were two of the "suits" on the grassy field that windy afternoon. We had been involved at the Smithville site off and on for some years; in John's case, since the problem was first recognized. We were there as members of Ted O'Neill's Strategic Advisory Committee. It was our job to provide advice on how to clean up the PCBs in the ground at Smithville.

There was only one problem. We didn't know how.

John and I peered across the field at the eight wellheads on the other side of the field. The wells had been installed some years before, in one of the earlier phases. The original idea had been to pump the oil out of the ground, just like Shell and Texaco do. So far, however, the wells had proven to be wonderful producers of water, but not very successful producers of oil. All together, over six years of operation they had pumped millions of gallons of water, but in all that water, only 250 gallons of PCB oils. We estimated that there were 8,000 gallons of PCBs still in the ground.

"So at that rate, we'd have to pump for a hundred years," I observed, "or maybe a thousand."

"Let's recommend that," said John; "the government would love us." I rolled my eyes. It had been made very clear to us that the government regarded Smithville as a politically disastrous money sink. They wanted out. The faster and cheaper the better.

"Well then, let's just turn off the pumps and walk away?" I suggested facetiously. "I mean, what would really happen?"

"Not much, I suppose. At least not much that really matters."

I wasn't prepared for such easy acquiescence. "Come on, John. These are PCBs. Polychlorinated biphenyls. Real live carcinogens. The big C and all that. The public would go ballistic if we tried to turn off those pumps."

"The public goes ballistic over any chemical with more than three syllables."

This was true, of course. The gaping chasm between public fears and "expert" assessments of the health risks associated with organic chemicals was a popular topic in our circles.

"Maybe we should bring in some toxicologists," I suggested.

John looked doubtful. In our hydrological and engineering fraternity, toxicologists are viewed a bit suspiciously. They seem hard to pin down. "Are PCBs dangerous?" we ask. "Well, on the one hand, yes. But on the other hand, no. It's all very complicated." They probably have similar doubts about us.

Our group headed over toward the treatment center, where the PCBs (and the solvents) are removed from the pumped water. My attention span was running out. Bigger issues poked their way into my mind. I turned to John. "*My* question is: What matters and what doesn't? Where does Smithville fit into the spectrum of human problems?"

John looked at me. "What do you mean? Scientifically, socially, economically, legally, ecologically, or politically?"

"Yes," I said.

John smiled ruefully.

By this time, our group was ambling back to the field office, ready to resume the advisory committee meeting. "So we either run the pumps forever, or we turn them off," I said. "Our hosts are not going to be too happy with us, if that's the best we can come up with."

John looked pensive. "Well, I guess they can just get in line then," he said. "The fact is that nobody's happy with us. And it's not just Smithville. It's all across North America; even more so in the U.S. than in Canada, with their Superfund laws, and all those lawyers getting rich. The corporations are angry because they're paying the bills and not getting much for their money. The politicians feel sandbagged because all their well-intentioned legislation hasn't solved the problem. Regulatory agencies are nervous because they're caught in the middle, unable to satisfy the conflicting expectations of politicians, environmentalists, industry, and the public at large. Developers are unhappy because the old environmental rules are out the window, and new rules are hard to come by. Mom-and-pop businesses that think of themselves as the backbone of America are getting fingered as environmental criminals just because they spill a little solvent out the back door. Environmental lobby groups can't decide who are the good guys and who are the bad guys, and don't know which way to jump to bring about positive change. Everybody is up in arms but nobody knows which way to shoot."

Our meeting started up again, then bogged down. We droned on, rehashing the health risks at the site, the costs and benefits of trying this or that, the uncertainties that beset us at every turn. I tuned out and began to muse on how we got into this mess. Overkill and underkill. Scientific uncertainty. Engineering infeasibility. Regulatory quagmire. What *do* we know, and what *don't* we know? What *does* matter, and what *doesn't?*

This book is the result.

1 The Polarization
of the Environment

For those of us old enough to remember, the birth of the environmental movement is linked nostalgically to the sensibilities of the sixties. To the middle-aged minds of many of us, these were the last of the really good times. There was peace and love. There were civil wrongs to be righted. In our memories, ideals drove our actions rather than selfish greed.

Or so it seemed. Perhaps we were just young.

Nostalgic memories do not always stand up to the light of historical truth, but in this case the timing at least is correct. It *was* in the midst of the social upheavals of the sixties that the first public awareness began to dawn that our consumer society was seriously fouling its own nest. Maybe this environmental awakening was aided by the tenor of the times, and maybe it wasn't. In retrospect, a period of social conscience may not have been a necessary element. The timing was perhaps inevitable.

A BRIEF HISTORY: FROM RACHEL CARSON
TO NEWT GINGRICH

The years leading up to and following World War II produced a chemical revolution that rivals the industrial revolution in its historical importance. It was based on research breakthroughs in organic chemistry that took place around the turn of the century. By the late thirties and early forties, spurred on by the war effort and the postwar economic boom, a deluge of new organic chemicals burst onto the market. These chemicals found uses in the new miracle drugs, in more effective solvents and adhesives, in dyes and paints and wood preservatives. They fueled the plastics revolution. They proved especially popular in the emerging electronics and aerospace industries. Synthetic organic chemical production in the United States was already 1 billion pounds in 1940. It reached 30 billion pounds by 1950, and 300 billion pounds by 1976.[1] Today there are more than 5 million chemicals known to humankind, 65,000 of them in commercial use, with more than 10,000 of these produced at greater than a million pounds per year.[2]

The early growth of this chemical society was not accompanied by a realization of the dangers associated with use and disposal of these new wonder chemicals. In retrospect, we can recognize the 1950s as an age of environmental carelessness. *Life* magazine called it the "throw-away society,"[3] but the editors of *Life* were probably more concerned with the perceived waste of resources than with the environmental impact of what was actually thrown away.

The bad news was bound to catch up with us. The age of Aquarius may have provided a receptive mood, but the facts were beginning to speak for themselves. Rachel Carson, the noted nature writer, fired the first round in 1962, provoking widespread public alarm with her attack on pesticide usage in the best-selling book *Silent Spring*. She emphasized the unintended ecological consequences of pesticide use and illustrated the interconnected web of life by reporting the presence of DDT residues in soils, plants, birds, fish, and animals the world over, even in such far-flung species as deep-sea squid and Antarctic penguins. Worse yet, she claimed, these "elixirs of death" were now stored in the body fat of human beings. They occurred in mother's milk and in the tissues of each unborn child. "It is ironic," she wrote, "to think that man might determine his own future by something so seemingly trivial as the choice of an insect spray."[4]

If the arguments of *Silent Spring* were a bit too nebulous and global for some, the growing number of specific contamination incidents that hit the headlines in the late sixties and early seventies were more concrete. These incidents involved individual tragedies with identifiable victims. Two incidents in Japan made worldwide headlines. In one, hundreds of cases of paralysis were traced to mercury poisoning caused by eating shellfish affected by releases from a chemical plant.[5] In the other, an unexpected rash of miscarriages was blamed on the use of rice-cooking oil contaminated with PCBs.[6] Closer to home, crop damage, sick livestock, and a variety of health complaints by farmers near Denver, Colorado, were traced to nerve gas by-products found in irrigation wells adjacent to the Rocky Mountain Arsenal of the U.S. Army Chemical Corps.[7] At the Stringfellow Acid Pits near Riverside, California, 32 million gallons of industrial effluent were stored in twenty lagoons in a canyon on the side of the Jurupa Mountains. When heavy rains threatened to overtop the retaining dam at the outlet of the canyon, National Guardsmen who had been called in for the emergency were forced to release 875,000 gallons of acidic wastewater laden with heavy metals, organic solvents, and pesticides down the gully, under a freeway, and into the Santa Ana River.[8] At Times Beach, Missouri, dioxin-laden wastes from chemical plants in St. Louis were mixed with used crankcase oil and spread on dirt roads for dust control. The citizens of Times Beach began getting sick. The government eventually bought all the properties in the community and permanently evacuated the residents.[9] At Woburn, Massachusetts, a cluster of leukemia cases in a suburban neighborhood was blamed on municipal well water contaminated by industrial waste. The court case that ensued became the subject of Jonathan Harr's book *A Civil Action*, which stayed near the top of the *New York Times* nonfiction best-seller list for more than a year, led to a popular movie starring John Travolta, and made this trial almost as famous as O. J. Simpson's.[10]

Of course the granddaddy of them all was the Love Canal,[11] which burst into public consciousness in August of 1977, with reports of black sludges bleeding through basement walls in a suburban subdivision in Niagara Falls, New York. There were initial reports of benzene fumes in the kitchen, dead trees in the backyard, headaches, skin ailments, and respiratory discomfort; and later of dioxin and miscarriages and birth defects. The story struck a chord with the American public. It was featured on the *Today Show*, the *McNeil-Lehrer News Hour*, *Sixty Minutes*, and *Good Morning America*. ABC put together a television special called "The Killing Ground." President Jimmy Carter declared the subdivision an emergency disaster area. Ultimately the government paid for the evacuation of more than a thousand households at a cost of $30 million.

But it did not do so willingly, and the evacuation process was carried out piecemeal over three years in a climate of high tension, misinformation, and broken promises. On Monday, May 19, 1980, the Love Canal activists actually took two government representatives hostage overnight, until they received assurances that Washington would take action on their behalf.

The source of all this woe was one hundred thousand drums of chemical waste dumped into an abandoned canal by the Hooker Chemical and Plastics Corporation more than twenty-five years earlier, in the 1940s and 1950s. The "canal" had been part of the grandiose plans of a flamboyant entrepreneur named William T. Love back in the 1890s. He had envisaged a utopian metropolis fueled by cheap Niagara hydropower. The Love Canal was to be a power channel delivering water from the upper Niagara River to the penstocks of a downstream power station. Alas, Love's grasp outreached his cash, and the Love Canal was abandoned after only one mile had been constructed. Thus did Love's dream become Love's folly, and then Hooker's folly, and ultimately a household name across America.

Before Love Canal, before the Stringfellow Acid Pits, before any direct threat to the health and lives of individual Americans had come to light, life in the environmental movement had been simpler. On April 27, 1970, Earth Day brought two hundred thousand people to the Capitol Mall and involved the participation of more than 20 million people in two thousand communities across the nation.[12] Both houses of Congress adjourned for the day, and forty-two statehouses passed Earth Day resolutions.

In these early euphoric days of the movement, everyone was on board. Earth Day brought together people from all walks of life. It brought in the old-timers from the conservation movement who remained focused on wilderness preservation and wildlife protection. It brought in the nature lovers and outdoor recreation buffs. It also brought in long-haired, youthful newcomers who saw in the environmental movement another outlet for their counterculture protest against established institutions and values.[13] Most of these groups had little in common except for a somewhat naive, apolitical version of environmentalism. Other participants arrived via the consumerism movement, or because of concern over the energy crisis, or from the antinuclear movement, which had been energized by the nuclear fallout scares of the mid-1950s. Earth Day was conceived by Senator Gaylord Nelson of Wisconsin as an "environmental teach-in." It was agreed by all the organizers, young and old, that there would be no civil disobedience or violence; and as it happened, everyone lived up to this unlikely promise. Earth Day was flower power all the way.

Unfortunately, this harmony of ideals would not prevail. As long as environmentalism was a vague motherhood issue, people of all political stripes and from all sectors of society could hold hands together. But from 1980 onward, a vocal segment of the population, with the news about Love Canal and Three Mile Island ringing in their ears, demanded action. Environmental activists took the lead; politicians responded; and legislation emerged. With legislation comes regulation, and with regulation comes resistance. The tentative beginnings of an antienvironmental lobby saw light, and the seeds of the eventual environmental polarization of the public were sown.

Table 1 presents an historical environmental timetable that attempts to put all these events, concepts, and legislative responses into perspective. In fact, it puts them into two perspectives, both of them looking backward from the present day with perfect hindsight: one representing the perspective of an environmental activist, and one representing the

Table 1 An environmental timetable.

Decade	Environmental Perspective	Environmental Events	U.S. Federal Response	Administration	Environmental Concepts	Influential Books	New Right Perspective	Decade
1940s	Chemical Revolution			Truman		Leopold: *Sand County Almanac*	Chemical Revolution	1940s
1950s	Age of Carelessness			Eisenhower	Throwaway society		Age of Economic Prosperity	1950s
1960s	Age of Awakening		EPA established (1970)	Kennedy Johnson	Conservation, wilderness preservation	Carson: *Silent Spring*	Age of Social Upheaval	1960s
1970s	Age of Awareness and Action	Earth Day Love Canal	CWA, SDWA, TSCA, RCRA, PP list, NOR	Nixon Ford Carter	Limits to growth	Commoner: *The Closing Circle*	Age of Overreaction	1970s
1980s	Age of Disillusion	Three Mile Island	CERCLA HSWA SARA	Reagan Bush	Soft energy paths		Age of Vindication	1980s
1990s	Age of Reaction	Earth Summit in Rio	PPA	Clinton	Sustainable yield	Gore: *Earth in the Balance*	Age of Reason	1990s

CERCLA = Comprehensive Environmental Response, Compensation, and Liability Act; CWA = Clean Water Act; EPA = Environmental Protection Agency; HSWA = Hazardous and Solid Waste Amendments (to RCRA); NOR = National Organics Reconnaissance; PPA = Pollution Prevention Act; PP list = Priority Pollutant List; RCRA = Resource Conservation and Recovery Act; SARA = Superfund Amendments Reauthorization Act; SDWA = Safe Drinking Water Act; TSCA = Toxic Substances Control Act perspective of what is now loosely known as the "new right." For the environmentalist (on the left of Table 1), the decades play out from an Age of Carelessness in the fifties, through Awakening, Awareness, and Action in the sixties and seventies; followed, unfortunately, by the Disillusion of the eighties, when the ineffectiveness of some of the legislative solutions began to become apparent. The new-rightist (on the right of Table 1) sees the Economic Prosperity of the fifties threatened by the Social Upheavals of the sixties, leading to the Overreaction of the seventies. To this person, the problems of the eighties represent an Age of Vindication. In the 1990s, one person's Age of Reaction is another person's Age of Reason. Both chart the same swing of the environmental pendulum, but they see it through different eyes.

To any reasonable person, there is no doubt that some form of government intervention was needed in the 1970s to stem the tide of environmental degradation. Consider some of the statistics uncovered at that time and since. American industry produces on the order of 250 million tons of hazardous waste each year.[14] That's 1 ton of hazardous waste for every man, woman, and child in the nation. In a widely quoted calculation, it has been determined that the average *daily* production would fill the New Orleans Superdome four times. Much of this hazardous waste goes to more than 3,000 special treatment, storage, and disposal facilities across the country,[15] and some of these have already experienced environmental releases. In addition there are more than 1,600 closed facilities where the containment reliability is even more open to question. Worse yet, it is widely recognized that in past years much of this hazardous industrial waste never made it off the plant property. The Office of Technology Assessment has estimated that there may be as many as 150,000 closed industrial landfills across the country.[16] In addition, the Environmental Protection Agency has identified more than 25,000 waste lagoons and impoundments at 10,000 industrial sites, with 50 percent of them containing liquid wastes with potentially hazardous constituents, 70 percent of them unlined, and 95 percent of them unmonitored.[17] Then there is the issue of underground storage tanks, with more than 1 million of them nationwide. Between 1984 and 1987, a California tank registration program found that almost 30 percent of the identified tanks were leaking.[18] All in all, it has been estimated that as much as 4 percent of the U.S. population may be at risk from surface-water-borne contamination (more than 9 million people), and as much as 10 percent of the U.S. population may be at risk from groundwater-borne contamination (more than 24 million people).[19] The U.S. Public Health Service has estimated that between 9 percent and 34 percent of the water-supply sources in the country are contaminated with the solvent trichloroethylene.[20]

With all these alarming facts in hand, the federal government swung into legislative action (Table 1). The Environmental Protection Agency (EPA) was established in 1970. The Clean Water Act, the Safe Drinking Water Act, and the Toxic Substances Control Act provided some early legislative response, but the real action began in 1976 with the passage of the Resource Conservation and Recovery Act (RCRA, pronounced *reck-ra*), and continued in 1980 with the passage of the Comprehensive Environmental Response, Compensation, and Liability Act (CERCLA, but known to one and all as the Superfund). RCRA put into place a government-regulated cradle-to-grave system for the control of all currently generated municipal solid waste and industrial hazardous waste. Later amendments to RCRA expanded the coverage to include underground storage tanks. The Superfund law targeted the legacy of past waste-disposal practices. It mandated the identification and cleanup of the thousands of sites across the nation that were seriously contaminated from inappropriate past activities. It was to be funded by a tax on the chemical industry, and it contains extensive provisions for cost recovery from potentially responsible parties.

The administration of these laws by the Environmental Protection Agency represents a major intrusion by the federal government into the lives of corporate America. From the beginning, the EPA has been under intense pressure: from the environmental lobby, on the one hand, to be tough and vindictive with corporate polluters; and from industry, on the other hand, to go slowly and be cognizant of corporate economic constraints. The two parties have seldom been happy.

In 1978, the EPA was taken to court by a set of environmentally concerned plaintiffs (including the Natural Resources Defense Council, the Environmental Defense Fund, the National Audubon Society, and others), who felt that the EPA was moving too slowly. The agency was forced to sign a consent decree with the plaintiffs in which it was agreed that the EPA would establish a Priority Pollutants List within a relatively short, fixed schedule. This list would identify, once and for all, the suite of chemicals that pose a threat to human health. It would insure that the EPA would give priority to these chemicals in its environmental protection programs. When the list appeared in 1979, it established 129 chemicals as priority pollutants, 114 of them organic chemicals, and most of these, synthetic organics from the chemical revolution. Under further environmental pressure, the EPA also established acceptable standards for many of the priority pollutants, in the form of maximum allowable concentrations in water.

Each of these determinations sent shock waves through the affected industries. An EPA listing could potentially end the demand for a particular chemical, as customers scurried to the alternatives served up by competitors, some probably just as hazardous but not yet on the list. Lobbying was intense. The maximum contaminant levels (MCLs) established by the EPA were especially controversial, and remain so to this day. There is no question that there are potential health effects from *acute* exposures to most of the chemicals on the Priority Pollutants List. Accidents in the workplace, experiments on laboratory animals, and limited epidemiology studies on humans have shown the impact of high doses. Many of the heavy metals, chlorinated solvents, pesticides, and petroleum hydrocarbons on the list are known or suspected carcinogens linked to cancer of the liver, kidneys, stomach, and lungs. Several are thought to damage the central nervous system, and others are known to damage the reproductive system, causing miscarriages and birth defects.[21] Acute exposure to trichloroethylene, which has apparently become so common in U.S. water supplies, can cause rashes, headaches, dizziness, nausea, and numbness of the face and hands.

What is less clear is the impact on human health of much longer exposures (over a lifetime) to much lower doses (orders of magnitude lower) of these chemicals. As the EPA struggled to come up with "maximum allowable" numbers, industry hollered that these standards were too tough, and environmentalists hollered that they were too lenient.

But all that was twenty years ago. With RCRA now part of the accepted industrial regulatory climate, with almost two decades of the Superfund under our belts, surely now we can look up and see the fruits of our youthful idealism. Do we have a demonstrably cleaner environment now than we did in 1970? Well, maybe yes, maybe no; as usual, it depends on who you ask; but nobody can deny that results have been mixed at best.

The question of greater political import these days seems to be: Can we see the end of the tunnel with respect to the current massive cleanup expenditures? Costs at Superfund sites seldom come in at less than $10 million; often they are many times higher. Total cost estimates for the Superfund program run as high as $100 billion. One estimate for the total cost of remediating *all* sites in America—Superfund sites, RCRA sites, military sites, state-mandated cleanups, and underground storage tanks—produced the sobering figure of $750 billion over the next thirty years.[22] These numbers are setting off alarm bells all over the country. There is no question that the nineties have been the decade of the backlash. Public interest in environmental matters appears to be waning. Embattled regulators are reduced to rearguard actions. An antienvironmental lobby has grown up that views the environmental movement as antitechnology, anti-free-enterprise, and downright un-American. This reactionary viewpoint was born in the environmental skirmishes of the Reagan administration, and reached maturity under the auspices of Newt Gingrich's Contract with America.

In a recent conversation at an environmental conference, one of the researchers from a right-wing think tank expressed his opinion to me that the real goal of the environmental movement is to bring down the capitalist system. In my view this is patently ridiculous, but cynicism runs high these days and conspiracy theories are in vogue, so I suppose there are people out there who believe this.

The election of "new right" governments at the state level has had a strong impact on environmental regulation. I can state from my personal experience as a technical advisor at a large contaminated industrial site in northern New York State that the instructions coming down the pipe from the offices of then–newly elected Governor George Pataki caused an abrupt change in climate at meetings between the owners of the site and representatives of the New York State Department of Environmental Conservation. The attitudes expressed by the state with respect to enforcement of environmental regulations at the site, previously quite harsh and bound by the letter of the law, became notably softer and more cooperative. Some would see this as a good thing, a sign of a more mature regulatory approach; others would see it as a sellout to corporate interests. Whatever it signaled, this change in attitude may well have been in keeping with the wishes of the people of New York: in the 1996 election they turned down a $1.75 billion bond designed "to preserve, restore, and improve the environment."[23] Similar results, which apparently indicate a greater fear of increased taxes and increased deficits than of environmental degradation, have recently been recorded in many other local and state jurisdictions.

In the Canadian province of Ontario, the election of a conservative government was accompanied by a full-scale assault on environmental regulations. In his first nine months in office, the new premier, Michael Harris, eliminated the ban on municipal waste incineration, vetoed Toronto's clean air bylaw, disbanded all major environmental advisory committees, eliminated intervenor funding, opened up a large northern provincial park to logging and mining, terminated bonding requirements for mine reclamations, and even terminated the funding for local blue-box recycling programs. The result is that Ontario has recently been identified as the third-worst-polluting jurisdiction in North America (after Texas and Tennessee).[24]

As another measure of the pullback, the total value of criminal fines levied in the United States by the EPA under its environmental statutes has fallen from a maximum of $169 million in 1992 to $27 million in 1994 and $5 million in 1995.[25]

To members of the new right, and indeed to many people of more moderate political stripe, the environmental pullback is not cause for alarm, but rather a return to reason. There is even support for this point of view within some regulatory agencies. At the federal level, the Common Sense Initiative is attempting to develop a more cooperative relationship between industry and government in the development of pollution prevention strategies for specific industries. At the state level,

attempts are under way in some states to develop self-policing procedures for industries. In Illinois, the Clean Break program provides am-
nesty for environmental fines for some polluters who agree to work with
the state in implementing pollution prevention measures. The business
community is happier, but environmentalists worry that the pendulum
is swinging back much too far, much too fast.[26]

Despite these tentative flirtations across the cultural chasm, the two
camps generally remain on their separate islands, warily eyeing each
other, both armed (at least with cash) and dangerous, with government
caught in the middle and the rest of us sitting on our hands. The environmental section of your local library still has two long shelves, one
filled with environmental motherhood, planet Earth, and sustainable
yield; the other filled with apoplectic frustration against the environmental hordes and their snail-darter mentality.

THE HIGH GROUND IS IN THE MIDDLE

So where should a reasonable person stand?

Well, I believe that most of us have views that lie somewhere between
the extremes, and we keep a suspicious watch on whichever band appears to be marching toward power. On the one hand, we are worried
that the current backlash will wipe out the environmental gains of the
past, re-creating the very climate that got us into trouble in the first place.
We don't quite trust corporate America to keep its own house in order.
On the other hand, we suspect that some of the health scares have been
overblown. We worry that there may be overkill in the current legislative
frameworks, and that current efforts at environmental cleanup are going
to bankrupt the nation.

In the later chapters of this book, we will examine the controversy
over the role of environmental contamination in human health and try
to establish what matters and what doesn't. We will attempt to identify
some of the unpleasant truths about waste management and the remediation of contaminated sites. We will look at RCRA and the Superfund

to see how well they have worked and examine some of the complaints of the now-polarized parties.

Surely by now all the cards are on the table. It must be time for a balanced examination of the claims of both camps. In this book we will search out the truths that undoubtedly reside in both houses and try to find a pragmatic workable path toward environmental protection. I hope to convince you that there is a set of environmental goals desired by almost all of society: things like reduction of health risk, conservation of resources, preservation of wilderness, and protection of wildlife; and also that there is a set of constraints accepted by almost all of society (at least implicitly): things like a desire for economic security, unwillingness to give up auto travel, and recognition of the unavoidability of hazardous waste and our need to dispose of it.

Some environmental goals can probably be reached in their totality. Others can be approached but not reached. Still others are currently not feasible, due to economic or technical impracticability. Solutions in a democratic society ought to be societally optimal. We should not expect them to be maximal in terms of all environmental goals at the expense of all the economic constraints. Nor should we expect them to be maximal in terms of all the economic goals at the expense of all the environmental constraints. They should be optimal: the best we can do with what we have.

It is the thesis of this book that there are social costs involved with both overkill and underkill in our approach to environmental protection. Over the past few decades, the environmental pendulum has swung between the "Greenpeace" endpoint and the "Contract with America" endpoint, but neither of these endpoints is desirable or socially acceptable. There are unavoidable trade-offs between economic health and environmental health, and it is not possible in a democratic society to sweep either one of them under the rug. Our goal must be to develop a rational environmentalism that will stop the pendulum without selling out.

And here lies *my* problem. A call to arms to fight for the middle ground is hardly stirring. It would be much more fun to write a book railing against corporate criminals or environmental pinkos. So while there is real need for a commonsense middle position, there is significant difficulty in promoting it. I will do my best, but arguments for rationality, trade-offs, prioritization, and negotiation do not provide the same clarion call as do marches on Washington or Contracts with America.

My involvement in environmental matters has largely taken place in the United States and Canada, first as a research scientist in the hydrological research community, and then as a consulting engineer on many RCRA and Superfund sites. In this latter role, I, like most consultants, have worked both sides of the street. I have consulted to the EPA and I have consulted to Eastman Kodak. (Cynics would call us technical mercenaries, but we still hold to the quaint view that technical facts are value-free.) This supposedly neutral role allows one to see both perspectives. I have listened to the regulators whine about the intransigence of the corporations, and I have listened to the corporate representatives whine about the unreasonableness of the regulators. What I have come to realize through all this whining is that there are very few black hats or white hats out there. The adversarial environmental milieu of the 1990s is a sea of gray hats.

At the end of each of the chapters of this book there will be a bottom-line summary in the form of a set of bulleted items that attempt to highlight the "truths" uncovered in that chapter. The issues are identified without fear or favor. Some will please one camp and some will please the other. Some will please both camps, and some will please none. The point is that environmental policies must be compatible with these "truths," awkward as they may be, not with preordained, doctrinaire, ideological positions.

CONTAMINATED SITES, CONTAMINATED PLANET

There is a web of interconnected environmental issues of global concern, but this book deals with only one of those issues. Emphasis here is placed on environmental contamination of soils, groundwater aquifers, rivers, lakes, and water supplies by toxic chemicals from industrial sources. Of particular concern is the contamination that arises from industrial waste-management activities. This type of source leads to localized contamination that impacts individual people or individual neighborhoods. Our scale is that of contaminated sites rather than contaminated planet. Of course, in the long run, one leads to the other.

This emphasis on site-scale contamination is not meant to minimize the importance of the "big" environmental questions of global perspective, such as overpopulation, deforestation, ozone depletion, global warming, and the greenhouse effect. In their most recent *Warning to Humanity*, the Union of Concerned Scientists sounded an unprecedented alarm: "Human activities inflict harsh and often irreversible damage on the environment and on critical resources. If not checked, many of our current practices put at serious risk the future that we wish for human society and the plant and animal kingdom."[27] They point out that global food production is being outpaced by growth in consumption in many parts of the world; that destructive logging and deforestation practices are wreaking havoc on the world's remaining tropical forests, amplifying soil erosion and water wastage, and enhancing global warming; and that there is now a discernible human influence on global climate that is likely to lead to higher sea levels, threatening populations and ecosystems in coastal regions, and to the encroachment of tropical diseases upon higher latitudes. These issues deserve the attention of any thinking person, but they are not the subject of this book.

There *will* be discussions of national environmental priorities and where the cleanup of contaminated sites ought to fit into those priorities. Currently in North America, the amount of money spent on contaminated sites far outstrips that earmarked for the study of these global problems. It is reasonable to ask whether the present legislative and regulatory emphasis on site-scale activities is appropriate, or whether global-scale issues deserve greater funding. Under current political realities, with deficit-busting and tax relief at the top of the agenda, it is clear that increased funding for global environmental issues could only come at the expense of reduced funding for the current site-based emphasis.

Localized contaminant sources can give rise to both air pollution and water pollution, but emphasis in this book will be on water pollution.

This decision arises by simple authorial prerogative, reflecting my own background and experience. I have worked for a lifetime on water quality issues; I have only passing knowledge of air pollution issues. I suspect that many of the points I raise about water pollution also apply to air pollution, but if so, this testimony will have to await an author with more firsthand knowledge. Air pollution will receive passing mention but will not be discussed in any detailed, systematic fashion.

Perhaps more contentious, at least in the eyes of many environmentalists, will be my decision to limit discussion in this book to those impacts of contamination that affect human health. I recognize, of course, that contamination also has impacts on natural flora and fauna, and in many cases these impacts are as important as the impacts on human health. Let me first make clear then that my decision does not imply that I think that the broader animal kingdom is somehow unimportant. Rather it is an attempt to keep some semblance of focus in the presentation. When risk assessments are carried out at contaminated sites, there are usually two very separate sets of calculations: one for impact on human health, and one for impact on ecological health. The toxicological profiles are very different, the water quality standards are very different, and the remedial actions that are likely to come under consideration may be very different, depending on which of these two exposure pathways is most critical. I fully support this duality. However, I have decided that trying to introduce all the technical concepts needed to support this duality would not be worthwhile. More pragmatically, it is clear to me that risk of human health degradation acts as the primary driver in the development of public environmental concern. For all these reasons, and recognizing that I risk some loss in appeal, I have elected to highlight human health at the expense of ecological health in the chapters that follow.

Lastly, I note that this book is written from a North American perspective. The United States and Canada are two of the most highly developed countries in the world, and two of the wealthiest. The types of problems discussed in this book are representative of those that occur in developed countries, and the steps being taken to try to solve them are representative of those being taken by wealthy countries. This perspective has resonance for only a very few countries in the world outside our own: Australia, New Zealand, Japan, and the nations of Western Europe; perhaps Israel and Korea and a few others. It is not applicable behind the former Iron Curtain, where the fall of Communism has left a legacy of environmental problems much more severe than those in North America, and where the social structure to address these problems is completely absent. It is probably not even applicable in newly developed nations like Spain and Portugal, where cases of industrial pollution are just now emerging and regulatory structures are not yet firmly in place, although I hope that the lessons of the North American experience might provide food for thought in these countries.

It is certainly not applicable to the developing nations of Central Asia and Africa. In his thought-provoking political travelogue *The Ends of the Earth*, Robert D. Kaplan describes a world of disintegrating nation-states, warring religious cultures, dwindling resources, and shocking environmental degradation.[28] In Cairo, there is no publicly funded garbage collection. To fill the gap, a Coptic sect known as *zabaleen* collect the garbage, sift through it for their living, and live in squalor among the mountains of refuse that they collect. It has been estimated that as many as 50 percent of the *zabaleen* children die before adulthood of malnutrition, disease, and pollution. On the outskirts of Istanbul, millions of squatters live in poverty and filth amid hills of garbage and factories belching black smoke. In Baku, on the shores of the Caspian Sea, unchecked petrochemical development has led to poisoning of the air, the soil, the water, and the beaches. Kaplan describes it as a "lunar landscape of tar and oil." It is not possible to reconcile these sordid stories of the third world with a pragmatic dialogue about environmental alternatives in the developed parts of the world.

ECONOMIC GROWTH, ENVIRONMENTAL DEGRADATION, AND HUMAN WELL-BEING

Having made the decision to zero in on human health as my environmental metric, perhaps the first question that should be asked is whether there really is evidence of a decline in human health in the years since the advent of the chemical revolution.

At first glance, it would seem that there is solid evidence to the contrary. Average life expectancy in the United States has been steadily rising ever since records were first kept in the mid-1800s. The average life lasted about 50 years or a little less in 1900, 60 or more in the 1940s, and 75 in the 1980s.[29] It may well hit 80 soon after the turn of the millennium. Between 1920 and 1985, average life expectancy increased at the rate of about four months per year.

At first blush these data would seem to argue against major chemical influences on human health. However, like all statistics, they must be examined carefully. Much of the apparent increase in longevity is due to a significant decrease in the infant mortality rate in recent decades. The infant mortality rate has been cut from 20 percent (200 deaths per 1,000 live births) in 1900, to little more than 1 percent (10.9 deaths per 1,000 live births) in 1983.[30] If you want to make it to age 50, the most important step is to make it to age 1; 95 percent of those who make it to 1 make it to 50.

The decrease in infant mortality, while important, does not account for all the observed increase in longevity. Of those who make it to 50, remaining life expectancy has still been going up at the rate of about one month per year.[31] Improvements in medical practice deserve some credit. Diseases like tuberculosis, pneumonia, and typhoid fever have been more or less eradicated—at least as killers—from the developed countries of the world. At the turn of the century, tuberculosis accounted for up to 25 percent of the deaths in the United States and was as dreaded then as cancer is now.

Leonard Sagan argues, in his perceptive book *The Health of Nations*, that improvements in human resistance to disease have been equally important.[32] These have been brought about by improvements in nutrition, maternal care, health education, and fitness.

Sagan also notes that further reductions in infant mortality rates are unlikely. If this projection is correct, then life expectancy can be expected to plateau over the coming decades. This anticipated reduction in the rate of growth of longevity has the potential to mask any possible negative impacts of environmental contamination. In other words, even if such impacts are occurring, it may not be possible for us to separate them from the infant mortality effects. It may be impossible to identify unequivocally the very impacts we desire to clarify.

Another way to assess the impact of the chemical revolution on health is to look at the situation on a disease-by-disease basis. In recent years, heart disease has accounted for 47 percent of all deaths, and cancer 22 percent.[33] (In case you're interested, there is a 2 percent chance that you will end your life in a motor vehicle accident, and a 1 percent chance that you'll be murdered.) Of course, people must die of something, and because people are living longer now it is necessary to use age-adjusted mortality rates to compare the current situation with that of the past. It turns out that the age-adjusted mortality rates for almost all diseases, except cancer, have been decreasing in recent years. As the exception, the rate for cancer has been rising slightly. Because many of the new organic chemicals that have been released into the environment in recent decades are known to be carcinogens, it has been argued that this slight rise in cancer mortality rates could be due to environmental degradation.

Once again, however, one must use caution in the interpretation of the statistics. If one looks at the mortality rates for different types of cancer, it turns out that most of them have actually been declining, just like other diseases. For example, there was a 20 percent decline in stomach cancer between 1974 and 1983.[34] The one counterexample, and the reason that cancer rates are increasing overall, is lung cancer, which increased 15 percent during the same period. This growth is undoubtedly due to smoking, which became increasingly popular in the war and postwar years, especially among young women. (It is too soon yet for the very recent decline in that popularity to have shown up in the cancer mortality statistics.) In a widely quoted study, two British researchers traced 25–40 percent of all cancers to tobacco.[35]

Even that is not the whole story, however. In a contemporaneous study, another researcher found that even if we remove the contribution of tobacco to cancer rates, we are still left with a very slight increase in cancer mortality.[36] He surmised that this could be a result of the "chemicalization" of the environment.

Yet another approach to the issue would be to compare life expectancy in developed countries, where there is wide usage of organic chemicals, with that in undeveloped countries, where there is little usage. However, this approach also founders on interpretive complications, due in part to the lack of data in the undeveloped countries, but also due to the sanitation issue. The wide availability of clean water supplies in the developed world reduces exposure to waterborne bacteria and viruses, a benefit not yet in view in many underdeveloped nations. The effect of squalor and poverty on health and life expectancy in much of the world confounds any attempt to compare industrialized and nonindustrialized countries. The simple fact is that the state of public health in industrialized countries is far superior to that in nonindustrialized countries; but this is true for a variety of reasons not directly related to the presence or absence of organic chemicals and environmental contamination.

So, in a global or national context, we are left with data that is inconclusive. We have some indication that the cancer rate is marching down a different path than that of other diseases, but we must be cognizant of the influence of the tobacco habit. We also know that there are organic chemicals being released into the environment that are carcinogens, and that more of them are being produced and used now than ever before. Given this latter fact, together with the unclear cancer data, I believe that it is reasonable and prudent to be concerned that environmental contamination may be contributing to the increased incidence of cancer.

However, this concern must be coupled with the realization that the effect to date is undoubtedly small, much smaller, for example, than the effect of smoking. In the study quoted earlier, 2 percent of all cancers were ascribed to "pollution."[37] This is a small but not insignificant value.

Lastly, we must recognize that the issue is not really whether *all* of our citizens are at risk from environmental degradation, but whether *some* of them are.[38] It is unlikely that Love Canal affected the health statistics of the nation, but it certainly affected the lives of those who lived nearby. Over the years, there has been a clear message from the American people that they don't want to be at individual risk from a Love Canal in their neighborhood, regardless what the overall population risk may be.

REALITY CHECK AT VILLE MERCIER:
BLACK HATS, WHITE HATS, AND GRAY HATS

So, these contaminated sites may pose some additional risk of cancer, arguably small, but not totally insignificant; there are tens of thousands of sites out there; and you have heard of only one or two, probably the Love Canal and maybe some nearby site that your local newspaper tried to turn into a Love Canal. What do the rest of these sites look like? What's their story?

Well, we obviously can't look at them all, so I will again use my author's prerogative and pick one to highlight. This site is in Canada rather than the United States, which allows me to postpone a detailed discussion of the complexities of the Superfund until later in the book. Nevertheless, I think it is fairly representative. It is probably bigger than most, smaller than some. It is a success story of sorts, because the current health hazard is apparently very low. However, it took twenty-five years of wrangling and false starts to get there, and it has cost a bundle. The villains in the story are naïveté, stupidity, and inefficiency, not outright malice. And the folly comes from all sides: as promised, a sea of gray hats.

The town of Ville Mercier is just south of Montreal in the province of Quebec in the French-speaking part of Canada. The area around the town is rural and agricultural, and local farmers take advantage of the good clay soil to grow vegetables not commonly grown this far north. The clay soil was once an ancient glacial lake bed, so the land is extremely flat. There is only one topographic feature in view, and therein lies our story. It is a north-south-trending ridge of sand and gravel about a half mile wide. During the forties and fifties, this ridge hosted several large gravel pits providing sand and gravel for the postwar construction boom in Montreal. By the late 1960s these pits had been abandoned, and they sat unused and unremarked.

Things were about to change. In 1968, the government of Quebec was trying to prod the private sector into opening a liquid-waste disposal operation for waste oils from the city of Montreal. A government agency carried out a hydrogeological study of the Ville Mercier gravel pits and declared them well suited for oil disposal operations. In the same year, the same agency issued a permit to a company named LaSalle Oil Carriers Incorporated to dispose of liquid wastes into the pits. For four years, from 1968 to 1972, the LaSalle tanker trucks lined up at Ville Mercier to empty their loads of refinery sludges, waste acids, spent solvents, paint residues, wood preservatives, unused pesticides, and other hazardous liquid wastes into the pits. Included in the releases were benzene, naphthalene, phenols, and a variety of solvents, most notably the ubiquitous trichloroethylene.

The water table is high in the gravel ridge at Ville Mercier, so the pits were half full of water as the waste oils slid down the banks into what LaSalle now called the waste "lagoons." Some of the waste liquids, like the benzenes and phenols, being lighter than water, floated on the surface; others, like the wood preservatives and solvents, being denser than water, sank to the bottom. Before long, the lagoons were layered like a bottle of Italian salad dressing. There was a floating layer of oils on the top, a water layer in the middle, and heavy sludges on the bottom. It was not a pretty sight. Nobody kept proper track of the volume of liquids released into the pits, but it was likely on the order of 20 million gallons in total. Nobody seemed to wonder what was happening to all this liquid, given that the pits were already half full of water at the start.

It all seems self-evident today. The higher liquid levels in the pits created a downward and outward hydraulic gradient that drove the liquids from the pits—oil and water alike—out into the surrounding sands and gravels. In fact, we now know that the downward migration of the heavier liquids was not much impeded by the sand and gravel. These liquids sank to the base of the gravels and entered the underlying bedrock formation. This relatively shallow fractured sandstone formation is the most widely used aquifer in the region. It hosts the groundwater flow system that provides the water supply to the numerous wells in the Ville Mercier area.

Unlike what occurred in many other sites, it didn't take long for the truth to come out. In 1971, just three years after the start of the disposal operations, eleven domestic wells, some over half a mile away from the pits, became coated with black, oily goop. The water in the wells was contaminated with chemicals common in waste oils. In 1972, the government revoked LaSalle's permit and closed the pits.

The period from 1972 to 1997 comprises a twenty-five-year history of remedial efforts at Ville Mercier, and the story is not over yet. In 1972, the government authorized funding on the order of $20 million to construct a pipeline to bring water from Montreal to the Ville Mercier area to replace the lost water supplies from the contaminated aquifer. In the same year, the government went back to the private sector again, inviting a company named Goodfellow Combustion Incorporated to purchase the land, set up an incinerator, remove the remaining liquid wastes from the pits, and incinerate them. In 1980, the government authorized a successor company, Tricil Incorporated, to remove the basal sludges from the pits and put them in a landfill to be built on the clay plain nearby. All these actions cost an additional several million. In 1982, the government passed a regulation restricting groundwater use in the large region around the pits now serviced by the pipeline. In 1984, it established a pump-and-treat system at a capital cost of some $10 million to try to remove the waste oils from the subsurface formations. This system continues to operate, at a cost of $1 million per year; but for reasons that will become clear later in this book, the system has never worked very well. The amount of contaminant mass that has been removed from the subsurface in more than ten years of pumping is an insignificant percentage of the total mass there, probably less than 1 percent. In addition, treatment has proven difficult, and it has often been necessary to release partially treated wastewater to a nearby surface stream. Some contamination of the stream has undoubtedly occurred, having arrived there sooner through human intervention than it would have by nature's.

By 1992, the site had probably gobbled up $50 million of the taxpayers' money and one could argue whether anything meaningful had yet been accomplished. The aquifer was still contaminated, groundwater use was still restricted, and the pump-and-treat system was not meeting its objectives. There *is* one positive claim that can be made, however, and that is that no adverse health effects have ever been documented at Ville Mercier, nor is there any apparent risk to the health of the current population. In addition, while the pump-and-treat system has not been effective in removing contaminant mass from the subsurface, it *has* been effective in restricting further migration of the contaminant plume in the aquifer. It is not clear whether an environmental activist would agree, but one could argue that the current delicate stability achieved at the site is a form of "solution."

This, however, was not the view of the feisty new government of Quebec. When the avowedly separatist Parti Quebecois gained power in Quebec, they did so as a people's party, and the new Minister of the Environment publicly promised to clean up the province's long-standing environmental liabilities, including Ville Mercier; *and* he promised to do so by forcing the owners of these sites to pay the costs. This came as a shock to Laidlaw Environmental Services Limited, an arm of the giant international waste-management firm, which had purchased the incinerator operations at Ville Mercier in 1984 and was now the owner of record. The minister made it clear that he intended to hold Laidlaw liable for site cleanup even though they had not been involved in the original disposal. He requested his staff to draw up plans for a program of excavation that would somehow remove every last speck of contamination at the site. The projected cost was $100 million. When Laidlaw refused to take action, the government sent out its own request for bids on the proposed excavation, declaring in the press that the cost would be borne by Laidlaw. In 1993, Laidlaw filed for a declaratory judgment by the courts as to who should pay.

This court case has never been settled, because in the meantime, both Laidlaw and the government established separate expert technical panels to provide them with advice, and both came to the same conclusion: that the proposed excavation was technically infeasible, economically unwise, and would probably create a greater health risk than leaving things be.

And that's where things stand at the time of writing. A "final" remediation is still under consideration, but the form it will take, or whether it will be undertaken at all, is still uncertain.

Ville Mercier is not a Chernobyl. No lives were lost. It is not even a Love Canal. No lives were disrupted beyond repair. But neither is it insignificant. It is a blot on the landscape and a continuing source of potential risk. The impacts of Ville Mercier are highly representative of many large contaminated sites. There is only one Chernobyl and only a few Love Canals, but there are lots of Ville Merciers. When you think of chemical releases into the environment and the risks associated with them, when you think of Superfund sites or potential contamination from poorly designed landfills, Ville Mercier is probably a realistic type of scenario to have in your mind.

So who wears the white hats in the Ville Mercier story? LaSalle Oil Carriers certainly can't qualify, and in any case they are long gone from the scene. The Ministry of the Environment, the supposed protectors of the public interest, can hardly make a claim, having been responsible for encouraging and permitting development of the site in the first place and then stirring up murky legal waters in the later stages. Laidlaw, although caught in the middle on the big question, has been charged and duly penalized at the site for other environmental transgressions. The press can make no claim: they acted as a mouthpiece for the politically motivated posturing of the minister, treating the case as a traditional good-guy/bad-guy story, without uncovering the original culpability of the government until long after public opinion was set. Perhaps the only viable candidates for white hats are the members of the Ville Mercier town council, which played the role of citizen's lobby in this case. The council opposed the original dumping of the waste in the pits, and actually took the government to court back in 1968 to disallow LaSalle's permit. They lost the case and the permits were granted.

Surely this tale of mismanagement can't be representative, you say. Well, unfortunately, it is. At site after site, one finds the same type of long, complex history, full of bad decisions, misspent dollars, political meddling, and legal conflict. The questions, however, are usually the same: What is the best remedial action from a technical perspective? What is the most socially acceptable remedial action? What is the most cost-effective remedial action? And who will pay for it?

THE ROLE OF THE MEDIA: SOUND BITES, MAVERICK SCIENTISTS, AND MAN BITES DOG

There is no question that media coverage of environmental issues has a huge impact on public perceptions and the resulting political response. It can be argued that the strict provisions of the Superfund legislation (almost vindictive in some aspects) were a direct outgrowth of the sensational nationwide press coverage of the Love Canal. The story hit a public nerve: families in distress, a corporate villain, and government bumbling. Michael Brown, the Niagara Falls reporter who broke the story and followed it through its many twists and turns, won the Pulitzer Prize for his coverage.

Fortunately or unfortunately, Love Canal became the model for reporting incidents of environmental contamination across the nation, not all of which merited the same level of sensational coverage. Conservative writers believe that this has led to unwarranted fear and anxiety in the public that borders on "chemophobia." They argue that the public is getting sicker from anxiety than they will ever get from environmental pollution.[39]

Simplistic headlines often use loaded words like "nuclear dump" or "toxic poisons" that are bound to inflame public passions. The media often focus on spectacular and expensive failures (as the Superfund is perceived by some), rather than local environmental successes like the reduction of smog in San Francisco, the return of aquatic life to the Potomac, or the threefold reduction of lead in water-supply reservoirs for Atlanta.[40] Sensational claims usually appear on the front page; balanced rebuttals, on the back pages.

The media also seem to favor good-guy/bad-guy stereotypes. They usually see the local environmental citizens' groups as the white hats, and the malicious corporate polluters as the black hats. There are lots of cases of environmental contamination where this is true. But there are lots where it is not. Some citizens' groups oppose rational solutions and obstruct actions that would benefit the environment. And there *are* some good corporate citizens. Every incident requires careful investigation of the motives of *all* the players. At Ville Mercier, the naive early press coverage probably prolonged the agony; it took the press far too long to get it right.

Some members of the technical community feel that the media are antiscience and antitechnology. However, objective academic studies of this issue generally conclude that an antiscience bias is not widespread.[41] Scientific coverage has certainly grown significantly over the years. The *New York Times* had six times as much coverage of water pollution issues in 1986 than they had in 1954.[42] Scientists welcome the increased coverage but are often aghast at how they are quoted in the press, claiming that their technical explanations have been mangled and all the assumptions and limitations of their studies lost in the shuffle. They tend to be offended if the coverage is not suitably laudatory, having been trained to believe that the rigors of their rational, data-based scientific method are somehow superior to the emotional, value-based perspectives of the press and public.

More defensibly, scientists are concerned that journalists pay so little attention to the credibility of their sources. When Iben Browning, a business consultant with no training in seismology, predicted that a major earthquake would hit New Madrid, Missouri, on December 3, 1990, reputable earth scientists were flabbergasted that the story was picked up by the national press.[43] Credentials seem to mean little to the media. In environmental articles, they often give equal weight to the opinion of reputable scientists and to scientific mavericks who hold extreme minority views and have little standing in their field. As noted by Jay Lehr, a provocative environmental writer: "Science is not like politics. Everything is not opinion. There are truths and incontrovertible facts."[44] On some topics, attempts to create a level playing field are misleading to the public.

The most serious charge against the media is that the level of scientific literacy in journalism has not kept pace with the need for informed coverage of modern-day issues. There is a dearth of true science reporters and a lack of scientific understanding on the part of news reporters, who are often asked to cover fast-breaking stories that may have an important technical component. Most environmental stories are local, and local reporters in particular tend not to be versed in science.

The issue is not so much in the details; even scientists from other fields don't necessarily understand the hydrologic, chemical, or toxicological details of a particular environmental event. Rather, it is the fundamental lack of understanding of how science operates that is at issue. It is the competitive system of grant selection, research funding, publication of papers, peer review, and the open forum for disagreement provided by conferences and symposia that gives scientific results their credibility. Scientists feel that journalists should learn how to tell the difference between this reputable brand of science and the less reputable brand that emanates from self-interested industry associations (and in some cases, from self-interested environmental lobby groups).

Even more important, they need a better understanding of the nature of the scientific method, wherein hypotheses are put forward, experiments are carried out to test the hypotheses, and results are put out for review by the scientific community. When these results point to clear cause-and-effect relationships (apples fall because of gravity), the press usually gets it right. However, the press has more difficulty differentiating between statistical correlations and cause-effect relationships. For instance, in the Woburn, Massachusetts, court case it was never established that the leukemia cluster observed there was *caused* by the consumption of contaminated well water. What *was* established is that the higher rate of incidence of leukemia in the well-water users was statistically significant relative to control groups from the general population. The press reported the causal relationship as fact, but correlations are not fact. There are many other correlations that might have turned out positive had they been carried out (against air pollution levels, diet, or genetic disposition, for example). Toxicologists equally as competent as those who carried out the Woburn study claim that all previous leukemia clusters that have been identified can be explained by statistical coincidence rather than environmental exposures.[45] At the trial, reputable scientists testified on both sides of the issue.

The Alar scare of 1989 is an even better example of widespread press coverage of a scientific result of questionable authenticity. The Natural Resources Defense Council (NRDC), an environmental lobby group, carried out an in-house study claiming that residues of the pesticide Alar in apples could cause cancer in children. Rather than having the study peer-reviewed and put through the usual checks and balances of the scientific system, the NRDC chose to give exclusive coverage to the TV program *Sixty Minutes*, and then released their report the next day. As a result, apples were pulled from grocers' shelves around the country, and the sale of apples was brought to a standstill. Subsequently, but without much public impact, the NRDC claims were studied by the scientific community and found to suffer from serious flaws and errors. The same year, the National Research Council, an arm of the National Academy of Sciences, released an exhaustive study of disease and diet. This study recommended that Americans eat more fruit and vegetables.[46]

Probably the most controversial press support for maverick scientists has come from the most hallowed news source of all, the *New York Times*. William Broad, a highly respected science writer, has published two articles in the *Times*, one on November 18, 1990, and one on March 5, 1995, that have seriously undermined the likelihood of public acceptance of the underground nuclear waste repository under investigation by the Department of Energy (DOE) at Yucca Mountain, Nevada. The question of whether such a repository will be effective and safe is a complex one; the facts are not all in yet, and it is not my intention to discuss the issues here in detail. The point I wish to make is that the two articles in question were each based on the claims of scientists who represent extreme minority opinions (almost singular opinions in both cases). In the first article, Broad highlighted the views of Jerry Szymanski, an internal DOE researcher, who claimed that Yucca Mountain was unsuitable as a repository site because it had experienced multiple saturations in the geologic past due to rising and falling groundwater tables. In the second article, Broad publicized the even more alarming views of Charles Bowman of the Los Alamos National Laboratories, who claimed to have identified the possibility of an underground nuclear explosion, should the waste be buried at Yucca Mountain. Both of these views were opposed by almost all other scientists in the proponents' own research agencies. The DOE subsequently spent millions of dollars in attempting to assess and rebut these media-fueled controversies.[47]

Most of these charges against the press—oversimplification, sensationalism, lack of attention to the credibility of sources, and scientific naïveté—are probably true; but in my opinion there is little to be gained by railing at the perceived irresponsibility of the press. The fact is that things are unlikely to change. The American media are driven by sales figures and rating-point incentives. Sensational stories sell; balanced technical arguments do not. The media look for environmental sex appeal. For an environmental twist on the "Man bites dog" syndrome, how about "Water witcher finds water where engineer failed," which is a story; whereas "Engineer finds water where water witcher failed" is not. We may as well accept the fact that the media are not likely to change their ways; attempts to set environmental policy will have to contend with sensational press coverage and the public perceptions and fears engendered by it.

THE PUBLIC: CYNICAL, ANTIESTABLISHMENT, STREET SMART, AND OFTEN WISE

Understanding environmental problems and assessing proposed environmental solutions requires some level of knowledge of science and technology. Most environmental studies receive input from geology, hydrology, chemistry, biology, toxicology, engineering, and many other disciplines. How much understanding of these scientific and technological issues can be expected on the part of the public? How much understanding can be expected on the part of our elected representatives? What is the level of scientific literacy on the street, and is it adequate to produce an informed electorate that will recognize sound environmental policies when they see them?

Initial thoughts on the subject are not too encouraging. What should we make of widespread belief in astrology, dowsing, exorcism, angels, and abduction by extraterrestrials? What of the results of a recent poll that indicated that 52 percent of U.S. adults think humans and dinosaurs coexisted?[48] Or that 28 percent believe that it's possible to communicate with the dead?[49] What about the recent growth in religious fundamentalism, which views much of science as anathema, rejecting such *scientific* fundamentalism as the age of the earth, the geological time scale, and Darwinian evolution? A recent survey in Australia reported that one out of eight university biology students believes in a literal interpretation of the Bible.[50] Pay attention, now; these were *biology* students!

In his book *Innumeracy*, John Allen Paulos decries the level of mathematical illiteracy in society.[51] As one example, he notes the tendency of the public to underestimate the likelihood of apparent coincidences. Is it really that remarkable that Kennedy's secretary was named Lincoln, and Lincoln's Kennedy? Most students are amazed to find two people in the same classroom with the same birthday, when in fact the probability of such an event is greater than 50 percent, even if there are as few as twenty-five people in the room. This tendency to underestimate coincidence probably leads many people to give more credence than is due to statistical correlations relating health effects and environmental contamination. This is not to deny that there are many highly significant correlations to which significant credence should be given. The point is that some statistical literacy is needed to make the judgment.

The effect of this public scientific naïveté is exacerbated by the fact that the issues surrounding environmental contamination have surfaced at a time of deepening public skepticism and distrust of corporate, political, and scientific authority. Fifteen minutes with Rush Limbaugh should convince you. The loss of trust in science is seen by some in the rising interest in occult practices and alternative medicine, and even in the failure of the O. J. Simpson jurors to pay much heed to the scientific evidence. An environmental example may be provided by the growth in consumption of bottled water. Americans drink 2.7 billion gallons of bottled water per year, a 15 percent increase since 1985, and it is now a $2 billion per year industry in America.[52] Apparently people do not switch to bottled water for its improved taste (believe it or not, a "taste study" has ascertained this).[53] Presumably they do it out of distrust for their water purveyor, to avoid perceived health risks associated with their tap water. If so, it is ironic, because in many jurisdictions bottled water is not subject to the same stringent regulations and water quality standards that apply to tap water.

Perhaps the strongest antiestablishment feelings are reserved for the nuclear industry. A recent survey asked people to provide words, thoughts, or images brought to mind by the phrase "underground nuclear waste repository."[54] The most common images were those of "danger," "death," and "pollution." No credit was given for the relatively cheap and effective power that produced the waste. It appears that there is pervasive dread, revulsion, and anger against all things nuclear. The general response of the nuclear industry is to dismiss these fears as irrational and rooted in misperceptions. However, others have suggested a more likely cause. This view holds that public nervousness over things nuclear is a measure of the loss of trust in the nuclear industry by the public in the years since World War II.[55] It began with misinformation provided by the old Atomic Energy Commission in the 1950s with respect to fallout from atmospheric nuclear tests, and it has been kept alive by the self-serving responses by the nuclear industry to the accidents at Three Mile Island and Chernobyl. Other writers have noted that the public has been left out of nuclear waste decision-making.[56] Almost nothing has been done to enlist the public in the siting process or to collaborate with the public in forging a solution. The few attempts that have been made have taken the form of propaganda designed to gain support for decisions already reached by the technical elite.

So we are left with a picture of the public as cynical and antiscience; or at least that is how the public is perceived by the technical community charged with the job of producing environmental solutions. I suspect that this view is only half right. The public *is* cynical and antiestablishment these days, a legacy I suppose of Vietnam, Watergate, Chernobyl, government promises not kept, and "expert" prevarications large and small. In my opinion, public trust will be regained not by transparent public relations campaigns but by an observable improvement in the integrity of the political, economic, and scientific elites, and reestablishment of a proper covenant with the people. Cynicism and loss of trust are indications of a widespread social disease that requires treatment of the source, not of the symptoms.

The second charge, that the public is antiscience, is probably just not true. I think that most people reading their astrological charts recognize that they are only having fun. Even those with fundamental religious beliefs seem to be able to keep science and faith separate, like those

Australian biology students must have done. Grassroots polls regularly show broad support for science. In the 1996 *Science and Engineering Indicators,* drafted under the guidance of the National Science Foundation, it is reported that 89 percent of the public claims to be "very interested" or "moderately interested" in science, 80 percent believe that science and technology make their lives "healthier, easier, and more comfortable," and 72 percent agree that the benefits of scientific research outweigh any harmful results. Americans love science; they just don't understand it.[57]

Scientists must also realize that technology is not omnipotent.[58] In environmental matters, science and technology cannot be expected to overrule economics, legal issues, public perceptions, and political realities. There is no higher authority that has somehow decreed that a cold, rational, scientific perspective is superior to a visceral, streetwise reaction. We must recognize the great balancing value of street smarts and common sense. Witness the public wisdom in the Ville Mercier case. As noted by some earlier environmental writers, "Most environmental decisions are not about science and numbers; they are about morality, and decency, and the health of family and friends."[59]

AMATEURS AND PROS: THE ENVIRONMENTAL MOVEMENT, THE ENVIRONMENTAL INDUSTRY, AND THE ENVIRONMENTAL ELITE

The roots of environmentalism lie in the hobbies of everyday Americans. Bird-watchers who enjoy their weekends by adding to their life lists began to worry about bird habitats and join the National Audubon Society to express their concern. Hunters and anglers began to worry about the health of wetlands and forests and join organizations like the National Wildlife Federation, the Wilderness Society, and Ducks Unlimited to try to gain a voice in land use debates. Hikers and climbers became active in the wilderness protection programs of the Sierra Club. These are all grassroots organizations whose concerned members are by and large amateurs, not pros. Most bird-watchers are not ornithologists; most rock climbers are not geologists.

For whatever nostalgic satisfaction it provides us, we have tried to keep alive this Thoreau-like image of environmentalism on Walden Pond. The sad fact is that "it just ain't so" anymore. Like most grassroots activities begun by amateurs, environmentalism has been hijacked by the pros. As amateur computer hackers gave way to professional Web site designers on the Internet, as the joyful chaos of sandlot baseball gave way to the structured competition of Little League, so too, has grassroots environmentalism given way to the professionals.

The press and public should probably know more than they do about the huge industry that has grown up in response to the environmental awakening. Environmental professionals now control all three of the main thrusts of this industry: the movement itself, the thriving corporate world of environmental consultants and remediation technology vendors, and the elite cadre of academic scientists and researchers who study environmental issues.

In the movement itself, the organizations that seem to create the most impact on government legislation and regulation are not the traditional participatory organizations, but rather the newer activist organizations like Greenpeace, the Natural Resources Defense Council, and the Environmental Defense Fund. These groups do not have to service member needs like the traditional organizations. They are administered by professional environmental lobbyists, and their primary purpose is to influence public policy. To be effective in this role, they require a continuing inflow of funds from the public; and to insure that this comes to pass, they must keep their name in the public eye through well-timed, well-organized self-promotional happenings. Greenpeace's antiwhaling, antisealing, and antinuclear adventures are the epitome. They received wide press coverage and succeeded in turning a small Canadian eco-group into a militant international lobby group of considerable power. This approach may be effective, but in most people's minds, by moving in this direction, the environmental movement has undoubtedly lost some of its shine.

Perhaps the most unanticipated outgrowth of the government's legislative and regulatory program has been the gradual development of a huge environmental industry. In 1995 the industry consisted of as many as thirty thousand mostly small-to-medium-sized companies, employing more than a million Americans, with total annual revenues of $180 billion.[60] These companies develop and market the vast array of equipment and services needed for the environmental retooling of corporate America: piping, pumps, drilling and trenching equipment, air-stripping towers, water treatment plants, landfill liners, chemical analytical services, geophysical instrumentation, and so on. Perhaps the most influential part of this industry is the environmental consulting sector, which was itself worth $10 billion by 1990.[61] This is the coterie of professional engineers, hydrogeologists, toxicologists, risk analysts, and scientists of many other stripes who assess contaminated sites and design the appropriate remedial activities. Their clients include the owners of the contaminated sites, as well as the regulatory agencies who require technical oversight in their enforcement activities. Not all the polluters are corporate; as we shall see, there are significant liabilities within the military and in the government itself.

Even more influential than the consultants are the scientists and researchers who have reaped the rewards of a massive infusion of research funding in the environmental sciences over the past two decades. Funding has come from increased environmental budgets in the traditional scientific funding agencies like the National Science Foundation, but also from new sources of funds made available by government regulatory agencies like the EPA, through the nuclear waste initiatives of the Department of Energy, from the military, and from corporate America itself. Programs have flourished in almost every science and engineering department at most major universities. There have also been major environmental research initiatives at government research agencies like the U.S. Geological Survey; at National Labs like those at Los Alamos and Berkeley; and at in-house corporate research centers like those run by IBM, General Motors, Shell Oil, and Westinghouse.

The role of the academic scientists and researchers who make up this environmental elite has been an uneasy one. Like their forerunners, the physicists of the Manhattan Project, they have been thrown into a political maelstrom for which they have neither training, nor in most cases, inclination. They are asked, on the one hand, to act as public servants, to aid in the drafting and enforcement of legislation; yet on the other hand, they are courted by large corporations to act as technical consultants and expert witnesses on their behalf. Neither the public nor the corporate sector is looking for the raw scientific facts that this elite has been trained to provide; whether they admit it or not, both groups are looking for hired guns with credibility, to promote their own agendas. Scientists find themselves open to many funding temptations and facing a host of ethical dilemmas. They become wary of the press and wary of the courts. Some retreat back to their ivory towers; others take the money and run.

After the heady growth of the seventies and eighties, the environmental industry and its academic research arm have both been strongly influenced by the backlash of the nineties. The industry as a whole still showed a 4 percent growth in revenues in 1995,[62] but some of the indicator sectors, like analytical services and remediation services, have already declined. Research money is drying up, job offers are down, and there is a general feeling that the glory days have passed. There is much talk that the industry will move from being a regulation-driven industry to being a market-driven one, but for all the conservative leanings of many of these environmental entrepreneurs, the mood is rueful.

WHO IS THE TRUE ENVIRONMENTALIST?

On a recent trip to the Niagara peninsula in southern Ontario, I passed a sign on the side of the road that read "No Toxic Waste Dumps in Niagara—or Anywhere!" The sign was professional in appearance, with lettering that was neat and legible from a considerable distance. The artwork was eye-catching: it featured a black skull-and-crossbones with red eyes.

The people who put up that sign undoubtedly think of themselves as environmentalists. But they are not. The first half of the sign, "No Toxic Waste Dumps in Niagara," is a classic example of a "Not In My Back Yard" attitude—the now familiar NIMBY syndrome. It is not an environmental argument; it is a selfish argument. Now, all of us are selfish to some degree, and most of us would probably fall prey to NIMBY thinking if a waste facility (or an airport, or a prison, or maybe even a new shopping mall) were proposed for *our* neighborhoods. It is not irrational, or undemocratic, or perhaps even immoral to want someone else to bear the risks of society rather than ourselves. The NIMBY issue is a difficult one to solve, and there will be more to say about it later in the book. For now, let's set it aside as a rational, selfish response to an unwanted burden. But let's not make any mistakes: Attempting to avoid risk, and trying to protect the value of the investment in your home and property, does not make you an environmentalist.

It was the second half of the sign on the Niagara roadside that really attracted my attention. "No Waste Dumps Anywhere!" Once again, we might all have such a wish, but it is an irrational wish. It has no more relevance to everyday life than a wish that we all be given a million dollars by the government or a guarantee of perpetual happiness. Waste is an integral part of human society and some of it is toxic. There is no doubt that per capita waste volumes can and should be reduced to the absolute minimum. No rational person would oppose the improved deployment of recycling programs and other waste-reduction measures; these are valid goals and espousal of them would support one's claim to being an environmentalist. However, opposition to all hazardous-waste facilities is not only irrational, it is antienvironmental. When environmental lobby groups are successful in blocking the siting of a new waste-management facility, they take away the public's right to have a properly designed facility to receive its toxic waste. This stance does not produce an end to the production of all toxic waste, as the proponents of the "No Toxic Dumps" movement might naively wish. Of course not. People still demand their medicines, their solvents, their treated wood, their fertilized crops, their electronics, and even their plastics. The real impact of this type of environmental activism is to force disposal of these toxic wastes into nonhazardous landfills ill-equipped to receive them. The overall impact is much worse, and it leads to more widespread environmental degradation than if a proper facility had been built to receive the waste.

The problem here is that the environmental movement has historically been a spiritual force rather than a pragmatic source of practical advice.

This spiritual role has been immensely valuable, and society owes a huge debt of gratitude to the early environmentalists. They are directly responsible for the growth in public awareness of the importance of environmental well-being. They alerted us to the need for careful stewardship of our fragile planet. They pushed for recognition of the limits to sustainable growth. They acted as a catalyst for change in industrial waste-management practices. And they demanded a strong regulatory presence to protect the public interest in environmental matters.

This has been an honorable battle, but to my mind it is a war now largely won. The environmental ethic is firmly in place in North American society. It is now accepted that there can be no social health without environmental health. It is time for the environmental movement to turn the corner and take the next steps. The help of environmentalists is needed in making the difficult decisions on how to effect the necessary changes in society to ensure environmental health. There is need now not only for spiritual leadership but also for pragmatic problem-solving that takes into account the economic and technical constraints.

David Suzuki, in his book *The Sacred Balance*, offers one of the clearest expositions of the spiritual side of the environmental ethic. He argues that we often ask the wrong questions. We should not base our social decision-making on questions like "How do we reduce the deficit?" but rather on questions like "What are the things in life that produce joy and happiness?"[63] Surely no thinking person could disagree with this. Yet it is difficult to avoid the conclusion that there is a trade-off between personal economic health and environmental health. How much of our hard-won income do we want to see go to the preservation and remediation of the environment? We can picture this trade-off as a wire, stretched tight, with Rachel Carson holding one end and Newt Gingrich the other. Each of us must find a comfortable place to perch. It is difficult because we are being asked to choose between two "goods." How does one balance personal economic well-being, a purely selfish motive, against an issue like public health and safety, which may have a personal component but also involves higher moral motives?

What is clear is that one's response to such trade-offs is highly value-laden. These personal values are determined in part by economic status and in part by personality and upbringing. The poor are less likely to worry about the snail darter, or perhaps even the pollution of future generations; the rich have the luxury to worry about these things. At a more primal level, one can differentiate between those people with libertarian values, which emphasize individual rights; those with egalitarian values, which favor the least well off in society; and those with utilitarian values, in which decisions are made to maximize the sum of individual utilities.[64] Newt Gingrich probably fits in the first group, Rachel Carson in the second, and most scientists and government regulators in the third.

One particularly value-laden issue revolves around the right of current generations to create risks for future generations. The egalitarian view is that irreversible actions affecting future generations should not be undertaken if their consequences would not be acceptable to current generations. In 1987, the World Commission on Environment and Development (the so-called Brundtland Commission) defined "sustainable development" as "development that meets the needs of the present without compromising the ability of future generations to meet their own needs."[65] More recently, a workshop set up to discuss this issue proposed some principles for intergenerational equity that featured a strong obligation to the future, but also some latitude to favor the present. Among the ideas put forward were the *precautionary principle* and the concept of a *rolling present*.[66] The precautionary principle is a two-part test that first asks: (1) Does a particular environmental insult impose potentially catastrophic risks on members of future generations? and then: (2) Can we take steps to reduce those risks without substantially compromising our own well-being? If the answer is yes to (1) and no to (2), then the project that would create the environmental insult should be abandoned. In the rolling present, the current generation has the responsibility to provide the next succeeding generation (but not necessarily any generations after that) with the skills, resources, and opportunities to cope with any potential problems bequeathed to them. The issue of what kinds of environmental risk we are passing on to future generations will be a recurring theme in later chapters.

So, how does one identify the true environmentalist? Well, as I see it, true environmentalists are concerned by and responsive to environmental degradation. They feel compassion toward other species, other peoples, and other generations. They recognize the need for government regulation but would prefer more emphasis on foresight and planning for future prevention, rather than revenge for past sins. They prefer negotiation and cooperation rather than raw political power to solve environmental conflicts. They favor an open and participatory conflict-resolution environment. They recognize that decisions must be sensitive to economic realities. They accept the social consensus that both protection of the environment and economic development are important and compatible. They are aware of the environmental threats engendered by our millennial lifestyle with all of its material benefits, but they recognize the will of the people to maintain and improve upon this lifestyle. Lastly, they are willing to accept that wisdom requires at least two kinds of knowledge,[67] and that both may be necessary in the solving of environmental problems: scientific knowledge, which is measurable in time and space; and spiritual knowledge, which is unmeasurable in time and space, but which is still subject to evaluation. It includes those aspects of knowledge such as beauty, awe, reverence, and integrity.

THE BOTTOM LINE

- As a result of the chemical revolution, there are now more chemicals produced and used by society than ever before. Many of these chemicals are toxic or carcinogenic at acute doses, but their impact at low doses over long time frames is less well documented.

- There are tens of thousands of sites across the country that are contaminated with toxic chemicals. They are a legacy of past carelessness.

- In general, public health is improving, not deteriorating. Analyses of mortality statistics do not provide an unequivocal answer as to whether there has been any recent increase in cancer due to environmental degradation. It is possible that there has been an increase, but if so, the effect is small. The impact of contaminated sites is not so much an issue of national public health as it is an imposition of unacceptable risks on individual Americans.

- Most contaminated sites have a long, complex history, full of bad decisions, misspent dollars, and legal conflict. Good-guy/bad-guy stereotypes can be misleading; the actions and motivations of all the players at each environmental site should be judged on their merits.

- In deciding between alternative responses to environmental insults, it is proper to acknowledge strong obligation to future generations, but current philosophical thinking on intergenerational equity allows some latitude to favor the present.

- Environmental activists who oppose all new waste-management facilities are taking action that promotes, rather than curtails, environmental degradation.

- The media are not about to change their ways. Attempts to set environmental policy will have to contend with sensational press coverage and the public fears engendered by it.

- There has been a loss of trust on the part of the public toward authority, perhaps with good reason. This loss of trust has affected scientific credibility in environmental matters. Environmental scientists and engineers must recognize that most environmental decisions are not about numbers: they are value-laden moral decisions about the health of family and friends.

- We are currently in an age of reaction to environmental legislation and enforcement. There may have been good reason for the pendulum to swing in this direction, but there is real danger that it is going to swing too far, too fast. There are social costs involved with both overkill and underkill in environmental protection.

2 Blenders and Buicks

THE ENVIRONMENTAL CONSEQUENCES OF OUR ENGINEERED WAY OF LIFE

We'll start this chapter with a little game. Look around the room in which you are sitting, and identify five objects: a chair, the rug, the VCR, a bookshelf, the books on the bookshelf—whatever. Each of these objects represents a commercial product that you purchased because you wanted the product and you were willing to pay the price. I'm sure you don't think about it often, but the fabrication of each of these products required some raw materials, some energy, some water, and probably some chemicals; and somewhere along the way it probably produced a thimbleful or two of solid or liquid waste. In living our lives at the dawn of the twenty-first century, with all of our material blessings, each of us contributes in our own small way to the need for resource development, the demand for increased water supply, the pressures to create and use new organic chemicals, and the generation of liquid and solid waste.

There are those who would have us turn back the clock to simpler times, with no blenders, VCRs, or petrochemicals. But they are a minority, and theirs is an impossible dream. Most of us like this material life. We enjoy camcording our kids, and driving our four-by-fours, and micro-waving our popcorn. We are glad that there are opportunities to see the world through air travel. And we are glad that there are antibiotics and modern medical technology to keep us healthy into our old age. We are aware, of course, that there is a price to pay for all this high living, and that it comes in part in the form of environmental degradation. Therefore we also accept that among our societal obligations must be to identify and eliminate the unacceptable environmental impacts, and to minimize and control the acceptable ones. We long for environmental policies that will identify the available trade-offs, and maximize our life experience. For most of us, this life experience includes both a love of nature and a love of blenders.

PRODUCT CYCLES AND WASTE STREAMS

Let's return to the game. Suppose, for the sake of argument, that three of the five objects you picked were a book, a pair of scissors, and that vinyl raincoat hanging on the hook behind the closet door. Each of these products arrived on your retailer's shelf after a long chain of events known as the product cycle. Figure 1 illustrates in very general terms the product cycles for our three selected objects: one a paper product, one primarily metal, and one petrochemical. Human actions are in the square boxes; the materials that result at each stage of the product cycle are inside the circles. Raw materials are won from nature through drilling, mining, and harvesting. They are turned into bulk materials through refining, smelting, and milling. The bulk materials are processed into engineering materials, which are then used to design, fabricate, and market the products we use in everyday life.[1] At each stage of the product cycle, additional inputs are needed in the form of energy, water, chemicals, and other bulk materials; and at each stage of the cycle, liquid and solid wastes are generated. If we were trying to decide which of these

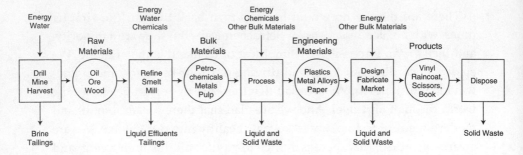

Figure 1. Product cycles for three selected products: a vinyl raincoat, scissors, and a book.

three products is the most environmentally friendly, we could not look only at the final disposal of the object after its life is done; we would have to also look at its contributions to the waste streams at all the other steps in the product cycle.

There is a movement within industry toward using this type of life-cycle analysis as a systematic means of evaluating and minimizing the environmental impact of products and processes. At each stage of Figure 1, the overall activity is broken down into its component operations, and for each operation the inputs and outputs are identified, with particular emphasis on contributions to air emissions, wastewater streams, and solid waste. The goals are to try to minimize resource utilization, energy consumption, and effluent emissions. Life-cycle analysis often identifies possible trade-offs between these goals in the form of alternative sources of raw materials, design alternatives, production modifications, or alternative waste-management options.[2]

Consider, as an example, the milling step in the pulp and paper industry. A pulp and paper mill takes in raw wood, adds water and chemicals, and produces pulp. Unfortunately it also produces liquid effluents that contain toxic organic by-products from the pulping and bleaching process.[3] These effluents have traditionally been released into the environment with little or no treatment. They have fouled many of the rivers and fiords along North America's West Coast from Oregon to British Columbia, and elsewhere around our nations. Environmentalists are rightfully upset, and, in part because of pressures from this direction, there is currently a strong effort in the forest industry to develop closed-cycle technologies that would eliminate pulp and paper effluents. This would be accomplished through wastewater treatment and recycling of the treated water back through the pulping process. Finland's pulp and paper industry has made a commitment to zero effluent status by the year 2005. The Canadian Pulp and Paper Association recently announced a five-year, $88 million program to develop closed-cycle technologies.[4] Similar efforts are under way with greater or lesser vigor in many other countries, and in other industries as well.

Only time will tell whether environmental pressures have been effective, and whether industry motivations are sufficient. Perhaps even more important is whether investors in these industries will accept the economic trade-offs. One of the unintended consequences of the mutual-fund craze that has swept across North America in recent years has been the spreading of ownership so widely and so impersonally that bottom-line economic performance can be sought by investors without apparent guilt. There is reason to worry that this investment climate may prevent companies from carrying out proper environmental measures based on life-cycle analysis without strong regulatory pressures.

FUEL CYCLES AND ENERGY ALTERNATIVES

The type of energy available for the production of goods has a considerable bearing on the environmental impacts generated, and on the health risks that must be borne by the population. Life-cycle analysis is well suited to the comparison of these alternative energy sources. In this case, the linked stream of processes like that shown in Figure 1 is usually called the fuel cycle. The nuclear fuel cycle, for example, is a six-step chain:[5] (1) *mining,* in which natural uranium ores are taken from the ground; (2) *milling,* in which the ore is mechanically and chemically processed; (3) *enrichment,* wherein the milled uranium is heated to form a gas and run through a gaseous diffusion plant in order to increase the proportion of the active isotope of uranium; (4) *fuel fabrication,* which involves the production of small ceramic pellets containing the uranium fuel, and their packing into fuel rods suitable for installation in a nuclear reactor; (5) *fissioning* of the fuel in the reactor to produce energy; and (6) *storage and disposal* of the radioactive wastes. Most proponents of nuclear power would like to see a *reprocessing* step before final disposal, at which time the used fuel rods would undergo a recycling step to capture additional available energy otherwise wasted. However, it is this step that leads to the production of plutonium in a form directly useful in the assembly of nuclear weapons, so opposition to reprocessing has been very strong, and up to this time, successful.

Radioactive waste is produced at all stages of the nuclear fuel cycle, not just in the reactor itself. It is usual to classify such waste as low-level waste or high-level waste on the basis of the strength of the radioactivity that emanates from it. In close quarters, low-level waste is dangerous; high-level waste is deadly. Low-level wastes include the tailings from mining and milling operations, contaminated solid trash from enrichment and fabrication plants, and outflows from the cooling-water cycles at the reactors. High-level waste consists of the spent fuel rods from the reactors. It is the high-level waste that is being considered for disposal in the nuclear waste repository currently being investigated at Yucca Mountain, Nevada.

During the early years of the nuclear power industry, several fuel-cycle studies were carried out to compare the costs, benefits, and risks of coal-fired power generation and nuclear power generation.[6] The fuel cycle for coal is simpler than that for nuclear energy, but it has many of the same steps: mining, milling, fuel preparation, and energy production in a power plant. Straight cost comparisons, in terms of dollars per kilowatt-hour of power, always came down in favor of nuclear power, sometimes by a factor of almost two to one. Analyses of traditional environmental impacts like air and water pollution also suggest that nuclear power is the cleaner fuel. However, the real issue in most people's minds is not the costs or the benefits; it is the risks. Most people view coal-fired power as relatively benign, and nuclear power as a dangerous and risky venture. The objective of most of these early studies, I suspect, was to try to convince the public that its perceptions of the relative health risks of coal and nuclear power, when viewed across the entire fuel cycle, were incorrect. Table 2 summarizes the type of data put forward in the late seventies and early eighties comparing the health risks associated with the two power sources. The risks are separated into occupational health (health risk to the workers in the mines, mills, and processing plants) and public health (health risk to the person on the street from the presence of these fuel-cycle activities in the community). In Table 2 public-health risks are further divided into those associated with normal power-plant operation and those associated with a disastrous power-plant failure. One can see from the table that for normal power-plant operation, the impact on health is far greater from the coal cycle than from the nuclear cycle. Expected fatalities and reduced life spans from air pollution caused by coal-fired plants far exceed the radiation effects from nuclear plants. This conclusion is undoubtedly still valid today.

However, public fears of nuclear power, then and now, do not revolve around normal operations. They revolve around the potential consequences of a disastrous failure. Table 2 compares expert and layperson estimates from those pre-Chernobyl years. The two estimates differ by a hundredfold. The risk estimates of laypeople are one hundred times higher than those of experts, partly because they believe that the probability of an event is higher than do the experts, and partly because they believe that the consequences would be greater. The laypeople envisaged a worst-case disaster with 2,700,000 fatalities.

We now have the experience of Chernobyl in hand, and although it may be viewed as lacking in compassion to try to reduce so human a tragedy to mere numbers, we can at least look at the statistics to see what can be learned. The Chernobyl meltdown led to 31 direct fatalities,[7] on the order of one fatality per plant-year. So in fact, both sets of projections were quite conservative. However in this case, the use of direct fatalities is misleading. It will be years before we know the full impact of Chernobyl with respect to increased incidence of cancer and other diseases, long-term genetic effects, and overall influence on the life expectancy of the exposed population. More than 600,000 people have been classified as having been "significantly exposed" to Chernobyl radiation, and estimates of future additional cancer-related deaths range from 5,000 to

Table 2 Health-risk comparison for coal and nuclear fuel cycles.

Health Risk	Units[a]	Source[b]	COAL		NUCLEAR	
			Estimate	Main Cause	Estimate	Main Cause
Occupational health	person-years lost per plant year[c]	S	200	Mining accidents and miner health	20	Mining accidents and miner health
Public health (normal power-plant operation)	person-years lost per plant year	S	5000	Air pollution	4	Radiation
	fatalities per plant year	FF	2–25[d]	Air pollution	1	Radiation
Public health (disastrous power-plant failure)	fatalities per plant year (expert estimate)	FF	<1	No major public impact	10[e]	Core meltdown, radiation
	fatalities per plant year (layperson estimate)	S	<1[f]	No major public impact	>1000[f]	Core meltdown, radiation

[a] A 1,000-megawatt plant is assumed for both coal-fired and nuclear power plants. A plant of this size can service approximately half a million people.

[b] Sources of data used in table: S = Schwing (Richard C. Schwing, "Trade-Offs," in Societal Risk Assessment: How Safe Is Safe Enough? ed. Richard C. Schwing and Walter A. Albers Jr. [New York: Plenum Press, 1980], 129–41); FF = Ford Foundation (Nuclear Power: Issues and Choices [Cambridge, Mass.: Ballinger Publishing, 1977]).

[c] Includes losses due to incapacity and fatalities.

[d] Low estimate for low-sulfur coal; high estimate for high-sulfur coal, no scrubbers.

[e] Pre-Chernobyl.

[f] Assumes one disastrous failure in 20,000 plant-years of operation (e.g. 200 plants over 100 years). Actual estimates were 17,000 fatalities for each coal-plant disaster, 2,700,000 fatalities for each nuclear-plant disaster.

40,000.[8] The anguish of the event, in and of itself, has undoubtedly colored the life perspectives of the Ukrainian people forever. I believe that most people would consider the common occurrence of Chernobyl-type events an unacceptable price to pay for the benefits of nuclear power. Despite the results of studies that lead to statistics like those in Table 2, purporting to show the advantages of nuclear power, most of us feel that there is something different in kind about radioactive releases from reactor meltdowns.

Later in the book, I will try to convince you that nuclear waste disposal is not the issue. There is no real technical impediment to the safe disposal of nuclear waste. It is not the waste end of the nuclear fuel cycle that poses the hazards to humankind; it is the reactors themselves and their vulnerability to meltdowns caused by human error, terrorist attacks, and acts of war. If you believe that future core meltdowns for any of these reasons will be sufficiently rare that they will not significantly impact human happiness, then there is good reason to support nuclear power as a viable energy alternative. If you believe that such failures could become common, then you have identified one of those unacceptable environmental impacts that ought to influence your stance on energy policy.

Regardless of one's philosophical views in this regard, it must be recognized that nuclear power is already well entrenched in North America's energy mix. There are 107 functioning nuclear power plants in the United States, and nuclear power accounts for about 20 percent of all the electrical power generated in the nation. (Coal-fired generating plants still carry the bulk of the load, with smaller contributions from hydro power and biomass combustion.) In specific jurisdictions elsewhere in the world, including Sweden, France, and the province of Ontario in Canada, nuclear power is responsible for greater than 50 percent of electrical power production. A pullback from this position, if such were desirable, would create a major dislocation in these nations' economies and would have to be phased over many years.

Largely because of Three Mile Island and Chernobyl, the nuclear industry is effectively on hold worldwide. Current reactors continue to generate power, but few new reactors are being built. Certainly, the heady early projections of a nuclear-powered world are now dreams of the past. The current plateau is probably the most desirable outcome of these recent past events from a societal perspective. It will give the industry time to perfect its safety protocols, if such can be done; and it will give the public a longer record of performance on which to judge the acceptability of the risks. All things considered, it seems likely that nuclear power will remain part of our energy mix for many decades to come. Those who wish to oppose this projection can choose to put their efforts in that direction; but there is an even greater need for more of us to see whether it isn't possible to make this truly remarkable energy opportunity work. What is needed from this group is not activist opposition to all things nuclear, but activist pressure on the nuclear industry to face the very real risks that becloud the nuclear option and to open their technical and social deliberations to public scrutiny. There is some evidence that this message has been received by the industry in recent years, and that they are awaiting the fruits of more constructive public input, if we choose to give it.

Partly because of the nuclear uncertainties, there is considerable public interest in alternative energy sources that are "safe" and "environmentally friendly," such as tidal power, wind power, and solar power. Some of these, like tidal power and wind power, simply do not have the potential to provide a significant percentage of the world's power needs. They can and should be part of the mix, but they are not panaceas. Moreover, it is not clear why they are so beloved by so many environmental activists; the environmental impacts of these technologies are far from benign. Tidal power generation would involve hydraulic works on more or less the same scale as hydroelectric power generation, an option that certainly has not found favor with activists. Control of a bay or estuary for tidal-power generation will not be different in kind from control of rivers by hydroelectric dams. As for wind power, one need only take a quick trip through the windmill fields, near Tehachapi, California, that cover the hilltops for as far as the eye can see to get a feel for the impact of wind-generated power on the landscape. Solar power, of course, is a different breed of solution. Perhaps someday it *will* be a panacea, but at this stage, it is still a dream. Research and development are ongoing, and probably ought to be funded at higher levels than they are. However, as with energy produced by the tides and the winds, most solar production is not all that environmentally friendly either, often involving huge areas of solar panels and considerable industrial construction for heat storage and energy transmission.

In short, while assessments of nuclear power, and investigations of alternative energy sources, can and should continue, when it comes to realistic options for the foreseeable future we are largely stuck with what we have. The energy needs of the world are sufficiently acute that it will be difficult to abandon any one of the feasible technologies. There will always be a mix of energy sources, and we must learn to cope with the environmental consequences of all of them.

LIKE DEATH AND TAXES: THE INEVITABILITY OF WASTE

Waste is an unavoidable by-product of human life. We can classify it into human waste, which is taken away by our sewer system; household waste, which is taken away by our garbage collection system; and industrial waste, the out-of-sight, out-of-mind waste generated at each stage of the product cycle or fuel cycle of the products we use in everyday life. Some of these wastes are solid and some are liquid. Some are hazardous and some are nonhazardous.

Most of these terms are self-explanatory, but the term "hazardous," which has been used rather indiscriminately up until now, is not. What exactly is *hazardous waste?* Well, it turns out that there are as many legal definitions of hazardous waste as there are environmental statutes, and as many academic definitions as there are textbooks. However, the recurring elements of these definitions seem to be the following: (1) a hazardous waste can be any element, substance, compound, or mixture; (2) it can be liquid or solid; (3) it may reasonably be anticipated to cause death, disease, behavioral abnormalities, cancer, genetic mutation, physiological malfunction, or physical deformation in human beings; (4) the genesis of these toxic responses may be physical, chemical, or biological;

(5) the exposure pathway to the receptor may be through dermal contact, ingestion, or inhalation; (6) the source of the exposure may be the waste itself; or it may be air, soil, or water contaminated by the waste; or it may involve an indirect pathway through the food chain; and (7) the threat may come from improper treatment, storage, transportation, disposal, or management of the waste.

This concept of hazardous waste is purposefully biased toward human health. A broader environmental definition can be achieved by replacing the phrase "in human beings" in the third element above with the more encompassing phrase "in human beings or other living organisms." In this book, as noted earlier, I have chosen to emphasize human health impacts rather than broader environmental impacts.

Using a definition with the above elements, most wastes categorized as "hazardous" are so designated because of the presence of one or more of three main groups of environmental contaminants in the waste stream: organic chemicals, metals, or radionuclides. The bacteria and viruses associated with the human waste stream, which would certainly fit the definition, are not usually thought of as "hazardous," perhaps because of humankind's long familiarity with sanitation issues and sewage treatment. The radionuclide group is a special case, almost totally related to the nuclear fuel cycle and the waste streams from nuclear weapons production. This waste stream is small in volume but large in visibility. The first two groups—the organic chemicals and the metals— account for most hazardous waste. It is difficult to think of a common household product that would not have contributed to both of these hazardous-waste streams somewhere along its product cycle. Any of the three objects that I selected earlier—the book, the scissors, or the raincoat—would provide a case in point. Production of the book, for example, undoubtedly entailed chemical releases at the milling stage and metals at the printing stage.

Accurate statistics on hazardous-waste generation are difficult to come by, and there are significant variations in the numbers depending on the source. The following estimates represent a compendium of several recent sources,[9] but most are based either directly or indirectly on the Toxic Release Inventories put out every few years by the EPA. It appears that there is on the order of 250 million tons of hazardous waste produced in the United States each year. More than 90 percent of it is liquid wastewater; only 10 percent is solid waste. Interestingly, 98 percent of this waste is produced by just 2 percent of the generators. These are the large generators who produce more than 1,000 kilograms per month (the so-called metric ton, about 2,200 pounds), and who have to file records with the federal government under the RCRA regulations. There are tens of thousands of these large generators, with about 55 percent of them coming from the chemical industry, 20 percent from the metals industry, 5 percent from the petroleum industry, and 2 percent each from the textiles, plastics, electronics, and transportation industries.

The 2 percent of hazardous waste that isn't produced by the large generators comes from more than 250,000 small generators, who produce less than 1,000 kilograms per month. Many of them belong to the local service industries and may include your neighborhood dry cleaner, auto repair shop, and film processing service. Unfortunately, as we shall see, the problems created by small generators are not necessarily small.

In 1988, there were 51 large chemical companies listed in the Fortune 500. They controlled 85 to 90 percent of their market. Their profits in that year ran to $124 billion.[10] This comes out to about $1,100 profit for every ton of hazardous waste generated, or about 50 cents a pound.

Hazardous industrial waste is only a small proportion of the total load of all industrial waste, on the order of 5 to 20 percent. The uncertainty in this percentage arises from inconsistencies in the available database. For example, mine tailings, agricultural wastes, and oil-field brines, some of which are undoubtedly hazardous, are exempted from RCRA and its reporting requirements, so they seldom appear in statistical compilations generated by the federal government. Whether or not these wastes ought to be exempted from regulatory control is another question, one that probably tells us more about Washington politics than it does about volumes of hazardous waste.

Household waste is largely solid waste. It contains more than 50 percent paper products. Estimates of generation rates run from 2 to 8 pounds per person per day,[11] which leads to annual totals for the nation on the order of 200 million tons, including more than 40 billion bottles and 75 billion cans.[12] The total numbers are increasing each year, but that's because there are more people, not because individual people are generating more waste. Per capita generation rates are actually going down.[13] Household waste is thought to contain only 1 percent hazardous materials,[14] mostly in the form of used motor oil, old batteries, oven cleaners, paint thinners, and the like. However, because it follows a disposal track designed for nonhazardous waste, household waste can create environmental impacts that are much more serious than simple consideration of this percentage would suggest.

There are not all that many things that can be done with this huge amount of waste, regardless of whether it is hazardous or not. The basic options are to store it, burn it, bury it, or pile it up on the surface of the land. Storage can be small-scale, in the form of aboveground or belowground tanks and drums, or it can be large-scale, as with the specially designed facilities built to store PCBs. The burning of waste takes place in high-temperature incinerators. Examples of buried waste include deep-well injection of liquid waste and the proposed underground repositories for high-level nuclear waste. By far the majority of the waste is simply piled up in landfills, impoundments, tailings piles, and other types of land-based disposal.

Each of these waste disposal methods has the potential to burden the environment with contaminants. Incinerators now handle more than 15 percent of all municipal solid waste[15] and a much larger proportion of hazardous liquid industrial waste. (This may come as a surprise to some, but yes, liquids can be incinerated.) Incinerators, even when fitted with scrubbers and filters, still send metals, acids, and dioxins into the atmosphere. They also produce a solid residue called fly ash that is exempted from the provisions of RCRA and thus ends up in ordinary nonhazardous landfills, despite the fact that it contains lead, dioxin, and other contaminants. All the rest of the disposal technologies—landfills, impoundments, repositories, underground tanks, and deep-well injection—have the potential to contaminate subsurface groundwater supplies through the migration of leachates from the land-based waste sources down to the water table and into groundwater aquifers.

Current waste-management practices control and delay contaminant releases to the environment but they do not stop them. In the next few sections, I will review the nature of these controls, and examine why contaminant releases are allowed to occur. In doing so, I'll be looking primarily at the technical issues, but perhaps the real issue is economic rather than technical. As noted in a recent editorial in a technical journal, the current cost of municipal solid waste disposal comes out to a few cents per person per day.[16] The true cost of the disposal, if complete environmental protection were attempted, would be on the order of one dollar per person per day. By accepting the environmental releases, we are effectively passing on the difference in cost to succeeding generations.

ENGINEERING DESIGN: SAFETY FACTORS AND THE PROBABILITY OF FAILURE

Our lives are surrounded by technology. We are bombarded by advertisements for the latest gadgets: digital cameras, interactive Web sites, and cars that talk to us. There is something exciting and romantic about these technological developments, and we marvel at the creative energies that go into their genesis.

However, there is another type of technology that surrounds us, more prosaic to be sure, so commonplace that we seldom give it much thought or appreciation. It is the technology of everyday life: the transport systems, the electrical systems, the heating systems, and the water systems that make our lives more livable. These are the technologies that make clean water flow when you turn on your tap, and make the lights come on when you flip the switch. Mundane they may be, but these systems work because they have been well designed, and when they don't work it is usually because there has been a breakdown in the design process.

Design is the domain of the professional engineer. When you take off down the interstate toward the beach or the ski hill, there is engineering design at every turn. Literally. Corners are banked to suit the design speed. Curves are spiraled to ease your entry into them from a straightaway. The concrete under your tires is designed to withstand the heat or the frost or the acid-polluted air, or whatever your little corner of the world has to throw at it. Ditches are graded and culverts are sized to handle the maximum expected rainfall event in your area. When you go under an overpass, you can rest assured that the concrete pillars have the strength to hold up the overlying roadway, and that the crossbeams will take the loads and stresses of the heaviest traffic and the fiercest winds. At least they ought to, because that is how they have been designed.

Questions of design arise just as surely in the design of waste-management facilities as they do in the design of a highway overpass. There are, however, important differences. Most traditional engineered structures, like the highway overpass, are constructed of conventional materials, such as steel beams and concrete pillars. The design analyses for these traditional structures are carried out in terms of the usual engineering quantities such as loads and strengths, and there are hundreds of years of precedent in working with these quantities. More important, there is very little uncertainty in most cases as to the design loads that these structures will encounter during their lifetime, or the strengths of the beams or pillars that will bear the loads. Even when large uncertainties exist, the costs associated with overdesign are not that great, and engineers are usually able to afford a large safety margin. That is, they can design beams and pillars that are considerably stronger than is actually necessary to bear the anticipated loads. As a result, the probability that a highway overpass will fall down under the weight of too much traffic is extremely small. Failure of these traditional engineered facilities is highly unlikely.

When it comes to waste-management facilities, on the other hand, and we choose to manage our waste by burying it in repositories or piling it into landfills, we are entering a much more uncertain design climate. Many of the engineering materials—like polyethylene landfill liners and nuclear waste canisters—are quite unconventional, and there is little precedent by which to judge their likely performance. In addition, the performance of some of the components, such as the leachate collection systems associated with most landfills, depends on the properties of the subsurface soils and rocks, and there are very large uncertainties in these properties relative to the properties of more conventional engineering materials. Analyses cannot be carried out in terms of traditional loads and strengths; instead they must reconcile the disparate and uncertain concepts associated with leachate generation rates, groundwater flow paths, and chemical transport phenomena. The bases for such analyses are still emerging from the research laboratories. Lastly, there is the question of what constitutes a failure. When a highway overpass falls down, there is no doubt that a failure has occurred. But how does one confirm unequivocally that a landfill is successfully preventing contaminated leachates from entering the environment? Seepage may be small, or it may occur very slowly, but it might still be significant. Subsurface detection is difficult. Often, seepage events that lead to environmental contamination are not recognized until long after the fact. In general, the likelihood that a design will fail to meet its objectives is much higher for a waste management facility than for a traditional engineered structure.

Now, I know what you may be thinking. What's all this bafflegab about design objectives and chemical transport phenomena? This is a dump we're talking about, not a rocket to the moon. Well, maybe so, but in this day and age, even a dump can be a major engineering project. Consider at one extreme a nuclear waste repository, such as the one under consideration for high-level nuclear waste at Yucca Mountain, Nevada. A nuclear repository involves considerable surface construction and extensive subsurface workings. On the surface, there will be waste handling and processing facilities, facilities to handle and store the mined-out rock, and buildings to house administrative offices, security patrols, radiation monitoring laboratories, and computer facilities. There will be cooling ponds and equipment yards and parking lots. There will be warehouses and cafeterias and living quarters. The subsurface workings will extend to depths of a thousand feet or more below the surface and will resemble a large mine. There will be several shafts, one for people and equipment, one for waste delivery, and one for ventilation, at a minimum. There will be a network of drifts and adits that will serve as the underground transportation corridors to take the radioactive waste from the delivery shaft to the emplacement rooms. All the usual requirements of underground design and construction will come into play. Rock mechanics specialists will be required to assess rock strengths and design the safest layouts for the underground workings. Groundwater specialists will be required to predict water inflows and design the necessary pumping systems to remove them. Mining engineers will be required to recommend methods of shaft sinking and drift advance. Designs will be required for the underground electrical systems, transportation systems, communications systems, and computer control.

The heart of the repository will be the emplacement rooms, where cylindrical holes will be drilled into the rock to accept the waste. The emplacement concept involves an engineered system of multiple barriers. The spent fuel rods from the nuclear reactors will be embedded in glass or ceramic and then encased in a metal canister. The canisters will be lowered carefully into the holes, and then the holes will be backfilled with a clay buffer material. Once all the emplacement holes in a room are filled, the room will be backfilled with the crushed rock from the excavation process. The rooms, and ultimately the tunnels, adits, and shafts, will be sealed at various points by concrete plugs keyed into the host rock.

When set down in a few sentences like this, it all sounds very straightforward, but of course there are many unanswered design questions. Which metal alloys will produce the best canister material to withstand the corrosive environment expected at depth? Which types of clay buffer materials are most likely to absorb radioisotopes effectively? What type of concrete mix is best suited to the rock-water chemistry at depth? What temperatures can be expected from the heat generation that accompanies radioactive decay, and what will be its impact on the rock, on the groundwater, and on canister corrosion rates?

A landfill is certainly simpler in design than a nuclear waste repository, but there are many similarities. A landfill also involves multiple barriers, but here they are in the form of surface caps, basal liners, and leachate control systems. And there are still lots of outstanding design questions associated with each of these individual components, and with the performance of the entire system as a whole. How can we design surface caps that will withstand long-term erosion? What type of polyvinyl material will provide the best containment properties at the base of the landfill so as to funnel contaminated leachates to the leachate collection system? What drain spacings and pumping capacities are needed to guarantee effective leachate collection?

All of these design issues lead to uncertainty in the anticipated performance of these waste-management systems. To see how this uncertainty is taken into account, it will be necessary to look a little more closely at the engineering design process. I will introduce such concepts as the *safety factor, engineering reliability,* and the *probability of failure,* and I will clarify the relationship between technical factors and economic factors in engineering design.

The engineering design process has traditionally been seen in terms of the relationship between the *capacity* of an engineered component and the *load* it is expected to bear. For example, consider the beams in that highway overpass. In this case, the load results from the traffic moving across the overpass, and the capacity of the beam is its strength. If the maximum load anticipated from the traffic is 100 pounds per square inch, then the designer need only choose beams that have a strength greater than this load. The ratio of the capacity to the load (i.e., the capacity divided by the load) is known as the safety factor. It is common in engineering design to use safety factors on the order of 1.5 to 2. To insure a safety factor of 2, our beam designer would select a beam with a strength that is twice the expected load. The inference is that for a safety factor of 2, the structure is twice as strong as it need be.

This traditional approach to engineering design presupposes that both the load and the capacity are known with certainty. In reality, there may be considerable uncertainty associated with either or both of these terms. Consider, for example, the design of a leachate control system at a landfill. This involves the design of a network of drains under the landfill to collect the contaminated leachate that percolates out of the bottom of the fill after rainfall or snowmelt events. The design questions revolve around what size and spacing of drains are needed to ensure complete capture of all the leachate, and what pumping rate is needed to remove the collected leachate. In this case, we can view the rate of leachate generation as the load and the rate of leachate collection as the capacity. In the traditional approach, we would estimate the leachate generation rate to the best of our ability, assign a safety factor of, say, 2, and design the pumping capacity to be twice the leachate generation rate. Here, however, it is easy to see that there is considerable uncertainty in both load and capacity. Even if we had a perfect way to predict leachate generation rates from a known rainfall event (which we don't), we would still have considerable uncertainty as to the timing and intensity of future rainfall events. As for the pumping rate, unless we have a perfect understanding of how effectively the drains will catch all the leachate generated (which we don't), we will have uncertainty about whether the design pumping rate is achieving our desired goal of intercepting all the leachate.

One way to visualize the impact of these uncertainties is shown in Figure 2. The upper histogram graphically illustrates our best estimate of the probability of occurrence of different rates of leachate generation from a particular landfill. The most likely rate is 100 gallons per minute, and it has the highest probability of occurrence, but larger and smaller rates are also quite possible. The range of possibilities is thought to lie between 25 and 175 gallons per minute.

A similar histogram could be prepared to illustrate the probability that specific rates of leachate generation will be captured by the design pumping rate. With a safety factor of 2, the design pumping rate is 200 gallons per minute (twice the likely rate of leachate generation), but the actual rate of leachate capture is uncertain. There is some probability that we are capturing more or less than the design amount. With this second histogram in hand, we now have two histograms, one representing the load (the leachate generation rate) and one representing the capacity (the capture efficiency of the design pumping rate).

The lower part of figure 2 shows the two histograms (now smoothed into bell curves) side by side. The bell curve for the leachate generation rate is on the left, and that for the capture efficiency of the pumping system is on the right. The most important feature in Figure 2 is the small triangular shaded area in the center of the bottom figure. This is the area where the two curves overlap. It indicates a region where the load *exceeds* the capacity. Even though the pumping system has been designed with a safety factor of 2, there is still some probability that the

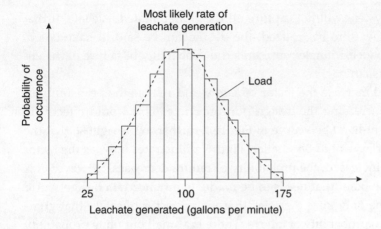

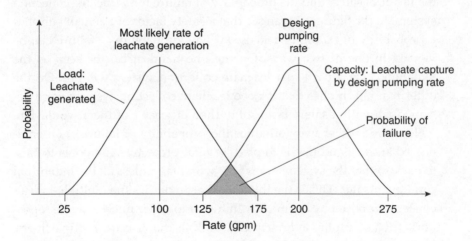

Figure 2. The concept of the probability of failure of a leachate control system at a landfill.

pumping system will not capture all the contaminated leachate. If that probability were to be realized, the design can be said to have failed. The little shaded triangle represents the probability of failure of the engineered system.

We could increase the factor of safety and reduce the probability of failure by increasing the design pumping rate. This would effectively shift the right-hand bell curve in Figure 2 further to the right so that the area of overlap would be smaller. Figure 3 illustrates how, as the factor of safety is increased, the probability of failure decreases. However, it is the converse point that needs to be made. In an uncertain design world (which is the only kind there is), there is no factor of safety that guarantees a zero probability of failure. There is a small but finite probability of failure associated with any traditional engineering factor of safety.

Let us assume that Figure 3 is representative of the relation between the factor of safety and the probability of failure for a leachate collection system. In the figure, one can see that a safety factor of 2 actually implies a probability of failure of 1 in 1,000. This probability of failure can be viewed in one of two ways. On the one hand, it can be seen as the likelihood that a particular leachate collection system will fail. On the other hand, it implies that if 1,000 leachate collection systems were designed, all with a safety factor of 2, then at least 1 of them would fail.

There is another way to reduce the probability of failure of an engineered system, and that is to place several protective components back to back so that the system as a whole won't fail unless all the individual components fail. This is the thinking that underlies the multiple-barrier concept proposed by the nuclear industry for their nuclear waste repositories. It also applies in principle to landfills that feature multiple liners, or liners in tandem with leachate collection systems. The probability of the serial failure of a system of components is held to be the product of their individual probabilities of failure. Two components with probabilities of failure of 1 in 1,000 lead to a system with a probability of failure of 1 in 1 million. That's the theory in any case, but as we shall see shortly, this much-vaunted multiplier effect can be very misleading. When it comes to long-term safety, we will be shooting it down in flames before the chapter is out.

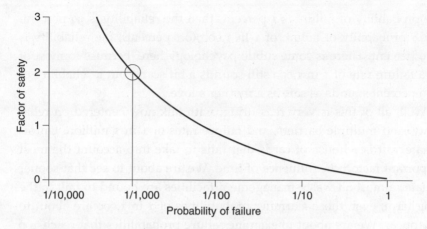

Figure 3. The relationship between the factor of safety and the probability of failure for a leachate collection system.

Most engineers who ply their trade in the more traditional branches of engineering would be aghast at mention of probabilities of failure as large as 1 in 1,000, even for individual components, let alone multiple-barrier systems. Highway overpasses, for example, almost never fall down. Their probability of failure is likely greater than 1 in 1 million. Large dams, on the other hand, which occupy a more uncertain niche in the engineering spectrum, have historically failed at a rate of about 1 in 10,000.[17] Every time dam engineers get ready to claim an improved safety rate, another dam gives way to bring them back in line. A projected failure rate of 1 in 1,000 may seem large, but it may not be out of line for environmental engineering projects, which are undoubtedly even more uncertain in their performance than dams.

While engineers may be aghast at probabilities of failure of 1 in 1,000, their clients are aghast at any mention of failure at all. The owners and operators of large engineered facilities want the public to hear about the great benefits to be bestowed upon it by their facility, not about how likely it is to fall down, or what the probability is that it will pollute the environment. To assuage these client fears, the engineering fraternity has invented the concept of *engineering reliability*. It certainly sounds better, but it is nothing more than the converse of the probability of failure. If the probability of failure is 1 percent, then the reliability is 99 percent. For a probability of failure of 1 in 1,000 (0.1 percent), the reliability is 99.9 percent. There is some subtle psychology here, because to most of us a failure rate of 1 in 1,000 still sounds a bit scary, but a reliability of 99.9 percent sounds as safe as a mother's love.

Well, all of this is very reassuring, with talk now centered on reliability, and multiple barriers, and failure rates of 1 in 1 million. Unfortunately, it is a house of cards that fails to take into account the most important factor: the influence of time. We are about to see that sooner or later almost all waste-management facilities are bound to fail. In the long term, even those alarming probabilities of 1 in 1,000 are about to disappear. We are about to examine failure probabilities that reach 100 percent.

THE LONGEVITY CATCH: HOW LONG DO THINGS LAST?

Things simply do not last forever. This certainly applies to human beings: we looked earlier at the expected life span for the human body and some of the causes of its mortality. In that discussion, we noted the tendency for the human mortality curve to exhibit an early peak that reflects infant mortality rates, and then a much later peak as the diseases of old age exact their toll.

The concept of a mortality curve is just as valid for each component of an engineered system as it is for the human body. Consider a landfill whose design includes only one protective feature: a single polyethylene liner installed at the base of the landfill prior to the delivery of waste. Let us define the *life* of this liner as the time between its installation and the moment when failure occurs. In this case, *failure* takes place when a leak in the liner allows the migration of contaminated leachate from the landfill into the underlying groundwater. Figure 4 illustrates a possible mortality curve for such a liner. Interestingly, it bears a strong resemblance to the mortality curve for human beings. There is a potential for early failures due to poor design, faulty materials, or inadequate instal-

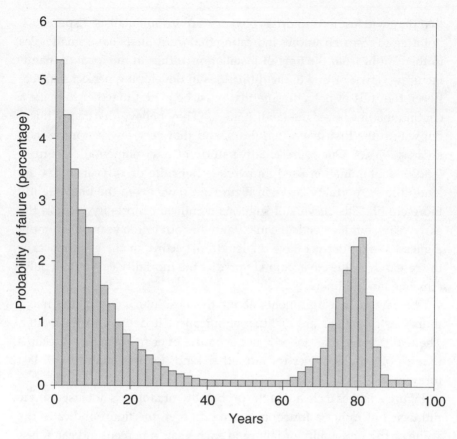

Figure 4.   Landfill liner mortality curve.

lation. If such failures are avoided, there is a good chance that the liner
will remain effective until it reaches old age. At that time deterioration
can be expected as a result of the physical and chemical breakdown of
the liner under the long-term effects of chemical interactions with the
waste, frost heave, burrowing animals, or any number of other potential
causes of damage.

The real question is: What constitutes "old age" for a landfill liner?
What is its expected life span? Unfortunately the technical community
doesn't yet know the answer to this question, and opinions vary widely
depending on their source.[18] The companies who make the liners claim

that they will last for hundreds of years. Environmentalists dispute this, pointing to research studies indicating that most liners have small holes in them right from the time of installation, either in the form of manufacturing flaws, or due to the difficulties in developing perfect seals between the rolls of polyethylene that must be joined together to make a continuous liner over the landfill area.[19] They believe that many liners fail within the first five or ten years, and that very few last more than about 50 years. One representative study of environmental risks from landfill contamination used an average liner life of 15 years.[20] On the landfill liner mortality curve in Figure 4, I have given the liner slightly more credit. This curve still suggests significant mortality rates in the early years, but it extends the maximum life out to 100 years. It is simply a guess. We do not yet have the length of record, or the experience, or the research studies to accurately predict the mortality curve for a polyethylene landfill liner.

The fact is that arguments about the absolute value of the maximum life of a liner are of little significance. It doesn't really matter. The real point is that nobody, not even the liner manufacturers, claims that a polyethylene liner (or any other kind, for that matter) will last forever.

Figure 4 makes it clear that the probability of failure is not just a single number, but rather a function of time. In fact, the figure indicates the value of the probability of failure in each year: 5 percent in year 1, less than 1 percent in years 40 to 60, about 3 percent in year 80. The total probability of failure over the liner lifetime is 100 percent. Just like people, the liners are bound to die. The only question is when.

The same arguments apply to leachate collection systems. They, too, have a finite life. One perhaps shorter than that of the liners, perhaps longer; but finite. Drains clog; pumping capacity declines with time; administrative control is lost. Whatever the reasons, they will not last forever.

At this point one might well ask if it is necessary that landfills last forever. Perhaps the worst contaminants are flushed out of the landfill in the first few years. Wouldn't one expect landfill leachates to become more benign as the years go by? Well, there is some evidence in this direction, and we will look at it in more detail in a later chapter, but the bottom line is that landfill leachates continue to deliver contaminants to the environment at unacceptable concentrations for periods that are much longer than the apparent life spans of the protective barriers.[21] We now have more than 100 years of record since the first municipal dumps were put in service, and because these early attempts at waste disposal were poorly sited and poorly designed, most of them leak. Many of these leaking sites still produce leachates that are highly charged with contaminants many decades after their closure.

In principle, nuclear wastes present a special case in this regard. After all, radioactive wastes are known to decay over time. Each radioactive isotope has a *half-life* that defines the time it takes for a given mass of the isotope to lose half its radioactive strength. Is it then possible to design a canister for a nuclear repository that would delay the release of the radioactivity until such time as its effect on human health would be benign? The question is not as simple as it looks, but once again the bottom-line answer appears to be no. During the radioactive decay of high-level waste, many radioactive isotopes of many different elements occur. Some of them decay to innocuous levels in a few hundred years, while others persist for hundreds of thousands of years. Some of the emissions from the long-lived isotopes are very harmful and some are less so. The safety analysis of nuclear waste is dominated by a few of these harmful, long-lived isotopes. After 1,000 years, even after 10,000 years, the radioactive releases would still be too hot to ignore.

When one hears engineers struggle with the concept of a design period for a nuclear repository, there seems to be a threshold beyond which even the most hard-headed engineer fears to venture. Some engineers get queasy at 100 years; many would be willing to discuss a time frame of 1,000 years; but 10,000 years is just too long. Even the nuclear-waste agencies themselves are hesitant to claim mortality curves for their canisters that exhibit life spans that exceed 1,000 years. I call it the "Giza rationale." After all, the pyramids at Giza were presumably designed by engineers. They were built with state-of-the-art technology. And they are still standing. They have been there longer than 1,000 years but less than 10,000. Even in this high-tech end of the waste-management world, there may be no better rationale.

Both the nuclear industry and landfill designers appear to place much stock in the multiple-barrier concept and its ability to reduce probabilities of failure through the compounding of reliabilities of multiple components in series. This reduction can certainly be achieved in the short term, but it cannot be sustained in the long term. Multiple barriers founder on the longevity catch just like single barriers. Consider Figure 5 where we compare the mortality curves for single-liner and double-liner systems. As expected, the probabilities of failure in the early years are much reduced. However, the life span of a two-liner system is no longer than that for a one-liner system, as all the liners would be expected to deteriorate at about the same time. If the total probability of failure must be 100 percent over the maximum 100-year life span, and failures are reduced during the early period, then they must be increased during a later period, as indicated in Figure 5. The real impact of a multiple-barrier system is not to reduce the total likelihood of failure but rather to postpone it several decades.

It is worth pondering whether such a postponement has value. As we shall see in the next section, postponement has great value to the owner-operators of waste-management facilities, and that is undoubtedly why it has proven so popular. The advantages from a societal perspective are more problematical. Certainly, postponing problems to later generations is advantageous to the current generation, which is thus relieved of the true cost of dealing with them. But this strategy raises ethical questions of intergenerational equity, questions that I noted in chapter 1 and will discuss further in later chapters.

For deep nuclear repositories, and to a lesser degree for surface-based waste-management facilities, regulatory points of compliance—in the form of monitoring wells or surface-water sampling locations—are often located at some distance from the containment facilities themselves. If a facility is considered to have failed only if and when it falls out of regulatory compliance, then one could argue that there is a second component that should be taken into account when considering the longevity of waste-management facilities. This second component is the travel time

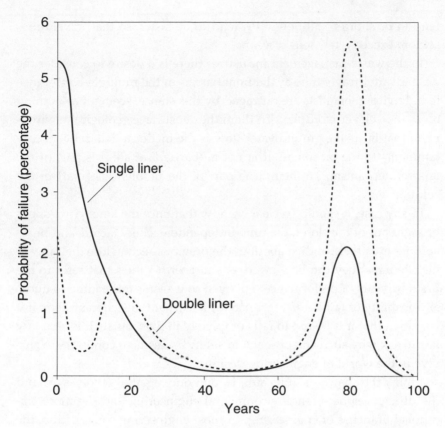

Figure 5. Comparison of mortality curves for single-liner and double-liner barrier systems.

for the contaminated leachates to be transported from the breach at the containment facility to the point of compliance. The usual mechanism of transport of the contaminants is in dissolved form in flowing ground-water, and as a result this second component has come to be known as the *groundwater travel time*. For nuclear waste facilities in particular, the distances from containment facilities to compliance points can be quite long, ranging from thousands of feet to a few miles. In some rock types groundwater flows very slowly, and travel times may encompass hundreds to thousands of years. For surface landfills, compliance distances tend to be shorter and flow rates tend to be faster, so that travel times seldom exceed a few tens of years.

In the waste-management industries there is a desire to consider the groundwater travel time as the final barrier in the multiple-barrier system. Environmentalists are outraged by this stance, seeing it as nothing more than clever wordplay. To them the subsurface geological environment that hosts the groundwater flow is the medium that delivers contaminants to the biosphere. It is not a "barrier" at all: it is part of the failure mechanism. To them, it is part of the problem, not part of the solution.

In any case, it should be clear by now that once the longevity issue is brought out of the closet, the time-independent safety factors and probabilities of failure bandied about in the previous section lose their meaning. Perhaps they can be viewed as short-term values that refer to the first few years of performance, but even so it seems misleading to quote a probability of failure of 1 in 1,000 for a leachate collection system, if it is known that it is bound to fail completely in due course. It is certainly fair to ask why such an approach to safety assessment continues to survive in the world of engineering design.

I think the answer is quite simple, and once again it revolves around the differences between environmental engineering and the more traditional branches of engineering. In most engineering construction, the idea of a project life is accepted and tacitly included in the analysis. It is understood that safety factors and probabilities of failure only apply over the specified life of a project. It wouldn't occur to the design engineer that a given safety factor would be required to hold up *forever*. It is anticipated that these traditional engineered facilities will be decommissioned or retooled when their life expires. Landfills and repositories, on the other hand, cannot be decommissioned or retooled. It is anticipated that they will be in place forever. One cannot envisage the wholesale reexcavation of buried waste, only to place it once again in a newly designed land-based facility, itself with a limited life. In cases where decommissioning or retooling are not anticipated, engineering design is a process of postponement—not prevention—of failure.

TIME HORIZONS AND DISCOUNT RATES

Time comes into play in yet another way in environmental decision-making: through the time value of money. To see the importance of this concept, we will have to abandon for the moment our societal perspective on environmental issues and instead think of things from the perspective of the owner of a new waste-management facility in the midst of the design process.

As the owner, you wish to construct a landfill on your site, and you have asked a consulting engineering firm to prepare some alternative designs for your consideration. The firm comes back with two possible alternatives. One involves a single liner; the other is a two-liner design. Both specify high-quality liner materials and tight control on installation procedures in order to reduce the probability of an early liner failure. Both alternatives call for polyethylene liners with a maximum life of 100 years. You must decide which alternative to construct. You listen to the technical arguments with interest, but you are a hard-headed business-person. The design process is not just a technical exercise, it is also an economic exercise. You do not make decisions on the basis of technical specifications; you make decisions on the basis of dollars. You are told that the double-liner option will cost $1 million more than the single-liner option. Your goal is to construct a safe, workable landfill at minimum cost and to realize a profit from its operation.

The economic comparison of engineering alternatives takes place in a decision analysis framework.[22] This framework requires the decision maker to assess the benefits, costs, and risks associated with each alternative. The benefits represent the direct income to the decision maker. As a landfill operator, your benefits will be the income you derive from your chargeout rate for waste disposal services. The costs are those associated with the construction and operation of the landfill. Both these components of your economic analysis are relatively straightforward. If you were to decide between the two alternatives based only on the benefits and costs, you would surely select the one-liner option. It costs $1 million less than the two-liner option, and the benefits will be the same in either case.

Why then should you even consider the two-liner option? It is because you hope that the additional cost may buy you some risk reduction. From the owner-operator's perspective, risk relates to the unwanted costs that would be associated with a premature failure of the facility. If neighboring lands or water supplies were to become contaminated, there would be cleanup costs to bear and perhaps regulatory penalties as well. There could be litigation costs to defend lawsuits brought by affected parties. There is almost certain to be some bad publicity and loss of goodwill in the community.

Like the benefits and costs, risk is measured in dollars. But unlike the benefits and costs, which are firm, the risk is probabilistic. The risk costs are borne only if there is a failure. Risk is therefore defined as the cost associated with failure multiplied by the probability of failure. Your engineering consultants will provide you with their estimates of the short-term probabilities of failure, perhaps 1 in 1,000 for the single-liner alternative, and 1 in 1 million for the double-liner alternative, as calculated earlier. It will be up to you to estimate the anticipated dollar consequences of such a failure. The probabilities are quite low, but the consequences could be great. In fact, it is not out of the question that the latter could put you out of business. In general, the larger the consequences of failure, the smaller is the acceptable probability of failure to the owner-operator, and the higher are the safety factors used by the engineering designers. In the case at hand, you may well feel that the extra million dollars for the second liner is worth the peace of mind.

In making these economic decisions, the owner-operator has a specific time horizon in mind. This is the period of time over which he or she hopes to recoup the investment and make a profit. The costs, benefits, and risks are not spread evenly across this time horizon. For example, there are up-front capital costs associated with construction, and benefits are obviously delayed until construction is complete and the facility can be brought on-line. The risks are also a function of time, with the probability of failure varying from year to year according to the dictates of the liner mortality curves, like those shown in Figures 4 and 5.

Economic decisions that involve dollars spent or earned at different points in time require consideration of the time value of money. Every investor knows that the value of a dollar won or lost now is greater than the value of a dollar won or lost sometime in the future. A dollar won now can be put in the bank and, with the interest gained on it, will be worth more when it is withdrawn at some future date. If you were to put $100 in the bank now at 10 percent interest, it would be worth $259 ten years from now. We say that the *net present value* (or NPV) of $259 gained ten years hence is $100. The 10 percent is the *discount rate* that allows us to discount future gains or losses to present value.

In your role as owner-operator it is logical that you should compare the single-liner and double-liner options on the basis of net present values. You will sum up the net present values of all future benefits and subtract from them the net present values of all future costs and risks. You will select the alternative that maximizes this sum.

There are at least two important implications of this decision-making framework. First of all, at discount rates that are on the order of current market interest rates, say 5–10 percent, the discounted value of all economic events that happen more than about 50 years in the future is essentially zero. Such events will have no impact on the owner-operator's decisions. Regardless of what the engineers may feel is their technical time horizon, the owner-operator's economic time horizon is less than 50 years. Second, it is now clear why the owner-operator favors alternatives that lead to the reduction of the probability of failure in early years and its postponement until later years. To an owner with an economic time horizon of 50 years, postponement of potential failure to 100 years is a worthy objective.

Discussion of these economic analyses should also clarify why there is need for environmental regulation. Left to their own devices, pressured by profit-hungry investors, and squeezed by competitive economic realities, corporate decision makers are unlikely to properly value the protection of the environment, especially on behalf of future generations. This role must fall to government. It is government's duty to carry out environmental protection from a societal perspective. The free-enterprise system is unlikely to do it on its own.

It is also worth noting that the monetary risk to the owner-operator does not include direct consideration of the health risk to the public or even the potential loss of human life. The owner-operator's calculations only take account of the dollar impact to the company's ledgers of such events, should they occur. The thorny issue of assigning a value to human life falls to the policymakers and regulatory agencies who must set the regulations. They do so, indirectly at least, when they decide on what level of safety to enforce. Increasing the required level of safety increases the costs that will have to be borne by the regulated industries, and these costs can be interpreted as dollars spent for lives saved.

Policymakers and regulatory agencies also require a decision framework in order to assess the merits of alternative policies.[23] They ought to identify the benefits, costs, and risks associated with each alternative policy, but now the benefits, costs, and risks are seen from a societal perspective rather than a corporate one. From this perspective, discount rates must be much smaller, perhaps on the order of 1–2 percent, or maybe even zero percent, in order to properly protect the interests of future generations.[24] In fact, there is a growing consensus that traditional discounting is simply not appropriate for intergenerational issues. This is especially true if the future environmental degradation involves health risks and potential loss of life. This view holds that it is inappropriate to use the same discount rate for money and for human life; the value of money varies with time, but the value of life does not. Most recent proposals argue for an approach in which lives and dollars are kept in separate accounts, and where monetary costs and benefits may be discounted but future health risks are not.[25]

What about the engineers who prepare the designs for waste-management facilities? Can't we count on them to protect public health and safety? We should, because the first fundamental canon in the Code of Ethics of the American Society of Civil Engineers states that engineers shall hold paramount the safety, health, and welfare of the public in the performance of their professional duties.[26] In the absence of regulations, I'm sure they would. The engineer would always prepare designs that are in keeping with his or her interpretation of the code of ethics. However, once a regulatory system has been put in place, it seems that most design engineers feel that they have satisfied their ethical obligations if they meet the regulatory requirements. They feel that the safety issue has been taken out of their hands, and they would find it extremely difficult to force their clients to exceed the level of safety mandated by the regulations. Regardless of whether this is a good development or bad (and opinions on this certainly differ), there is no question that this is the attitude that currently prevails in the nuclear-waste and hazardous-waste industries.[27]

In the design of waste-management facilities, there is an unavoidable trade-off between cost and safety. Facility owners will authorize only the degree of safety that reduces their own risk over their own relatively short time horizon. If there is a broad societal consensus that intergenerational environmental protection is in the public interest, then it is up to government to set regulatory environmental policies that will drive facility owners and their consulting engineers toward designs that feature greater safety, or perhaps better yet, more long-lived safety.

INDUSTRIAL OPERATIONS AND HUMAN ERROR: ACCIDENTS, SPILLS, AND LEAKS

Waste-management facilities are not the only sources of contaminant releases to the environment. Accidents, spills, and leaks occur daily at industrial plants across the country in the course of their normal operations. The potential for mishap lurks at every stage of the product cycle; misfortune waits at every step in the fuel cycles that drive industrial production. Accidents happen because of faulty equipment and poorly designed systems and administrative screwups. But mostly they occur due to simple human error. In fact it could be argued that the use of faulty equipment or faulty systems is itself a form of human error.

Picture a large industrial site, the kind you pass by on the smoky side of town. It may be a chemical plant or an oil refinery or a wood-treatment facility or an aerospace complex. Some of these plants are huge, with hundreds of buildings, thousands of employees, and an infrastructure of roads and parking lots and eating facilities and baseball diamonds similar in scope to that of a small city. There will be rail spurs and truck-loading bays and warehouses to handle the incoming materials of production. There will be laboratories that use chemicals, and machines that require petrofuels, and industrial degreasers that require solvents. The site will be a honeycomb of piping networks delivering process waters to the plant area and taking wastewaters away. There will be sewer systems and storm drainage systems. There will be pipelines and storage tanks for fuels and oils, and maybe for solvents and chemicals too.

This maze of support systems provides opportunities at every turn for something to go wrong: corroded pipes, faulty valves, broken seals, malfunctioning pumps, electrical breakdowns, warning lights that fail to warn, and response systems that fail to respond. There are taps that can be left open, barrels that can be dropped and broken. Human beings are not perfect. Some are lazy, some are stupid, some are impaired or hung over as they work. Some are just clumsy now and then. Meters can be misread, chemical samples can be mislabeled, hazardous waste can be dumped down the sewer by mistake.

Most industrial plants have strict protocols designed to prevent all these mistakes, and safety programs to try to cut down the number of accidents. These programs can reduce human error but they can't eliminate it. Usually the protocols include some type of "event" recording system to monitor plant safety performance. Most large industrial plants record hundreds of events each year, and many of these events involve chemical releases to the environment. I once asked the plant manager of a large chemical plant how many barrels of chemicals are lost in a year through spillage and leakage. He couldn't give me an exact answer, but it was clear that the number was in the tens of barrels or more (maybe much more), and that, in his opinion, reducing spillage to zero would be impossible.

What are the implications of this situation? Well, suppose for example that a fifty-five-gallon drum of trichloroethylene (TCE) were spilled on the ground and the TCE then infiltrated down to the water table. Concentrations of dissolved TCE in groundwater often run around one part per million. At this concentration, and assuming a subsurface porosity of 30 percent—which would be a reasonable value for a sand-and-gravel aquifer—this single barrel of TCE could create a contaminated plume in the groundwater that is 100 feet thick, 500 feet wide, and 2,000 feet long.

Larger spills and/or lower concentrations could create even larger plumes. For example, the regulatory standard for TCE is 5 parts per *billion*. In other words, if there is more than 5 grams of TCE (about a spoonful) dissolved in 5 billion grams of water (about 5 swimming pools full), then it is thought to be harmful to your health if you drink it. If that single barrel of TCE just happened to distribute itself throughout the aquifer at a concentration equal to the health standard, the resulting plume would be miles long! There are reasons why things are not quite this bad, and we will come to them in due course, but I hope the point is made. Even small spills can do much harm.

With these simple calculations in hand, it is not surprising that past operational spills and leaks have created highly contaminated soils and groundwater in the vicinity of most industrial plants. At some plants, hydrogeological conditions are such that the contamination has remained on-site; at others, contaminants have been carried far off-site by the flowing groundwater. The usual scenario features a long thin plume oriented away from the plant site in the direction of prevailing groundwater flow. If there are wells in the aquifer downstream from the plant, they will suck in this contaminated water. That is exactly what happened at Woburn, Massachusetts, leading to claims of leukemia in children, and the famous environmental lawsuit described by Jonathan Harr in *A Civil Action*.[28]

Human error seems to pop up at all stages of project development. At Ville Mercier, administrative errors at the planning stage of the project led to use of an inappropriate site for the disposal of hazardous liquid waste. At Chernobyl, operational errors led to the core meltdown that shocked the world. At the Hanford Nuclear Reservation near Richland, Washington, human error during a monitoring program caused a serious radioactive leak to go undetected for almost two months, turning what could have been an easily correctable problem into a nationwide cause célèbre.

The leak at Hanford occurred in June of 1973 from a forty-year-old buried tank built during the Manhattan Project as an "interim solution" for liquid radioactive waste storage. More than 115,000 gallons of high-level waste leaked into the ground, and the event received multipage coverage in both *Time* and *Newsweek*. The leak should not have gone undetected for so long. There was a monitoring system in place and measurements were taken on a regular schedule. One might ask, as an article in *Science* did, "How could they lose the equivalent of a railroad tank car full of radioactive liquid hot enough to boil itself for years on end and knock a Geiger counter offscale at a hundred paces?"[29] The National Academy of Sciences was asked to carry out an independent review.[30] It turned out that a key employee was on vacation in May and June of 1973 and his substitute had not been trained to recognize the signals. The lack of detection was attributed to "managerial laxity and human error."

The National Academy also concluded that while the event was indefensible, it had not led to any "significant radiation hazard to public health and safety." While this statement may have satisfied the technical community, public trust continued to be eroded by such events. In the March 28, 1983, issue of the *New Yorker*, the following brief item appeared:

Uh-Huh Department

(FROM THE *Vancouver Wash. Columbian*)

Richland, Wash. (AP)—Thousands of gallons of radioactive water are leaking from the N-reactor storage basin each day at the Hanford nuclear reservation, say officials.

They said the water is caught before it enters the ground.

"It may be going into the ground, but we are not sure," said a spokesman. "We don't think so. We are confident it's not."[31]

THE LEGACY OF PAST SINS

There is scarcely a community in North America that isn't host to one or more contaminated industrial sites. We have already mentioned the Stringfellow Acid Pits in Riverside, California; the Rocky Mountain Arsenal in Denver, Colorado; the Love Canal in Niagara Falls, New York;

and the Hanford Nuclear Reservation in Richland, Washington. We have looked at the Laidlaw site at Ville Mercier, Quebec, in detail and noted in passing the events at Times Beach, Missouri, and Woburn, Massachusetts. Figure 6 is a map of North America that indicates the locations of all these contaminated sites and many more that are going to be introduced in this section and throughout the rest of the book. As a random collection of dots, a blindfolded dart thrower could probably do no better.

I have already emphasized the leading role of landfills and other waste-management facilities as sources of environmental contamination, but one more story can't hurt. The Fresh Kills landfill, which serves New York City, is the granddaddy of all landfills. It covers four and a half square miles and is 505 feet high.[32] That makes it almost half as tall as the Empire State Building and more than a hundred times larger in volume. It is one of the largest structures ever constructed by human beings. When it is complete, it will be the highest point of land on the eastern seaboard.

The landfill was built in 1948 on a salt marsh on the west side of Staten Island. It has no bottom liner, and until 1994 it had no leachate collection system. It has been estimated that prior to 1994 the landfill delivered a million gallons of leachate *per day* into New York Harbor. A new leachate treatment plant now handles about one-fifth of the total leachate, and work is in progress to expand its capacity. Fresh Kills is scheduled to close in the year 2005. Regulations require continuation of the leachate collection system after closure, but only for thirty years. Leachate generation will continue forever.

Chemical plants are another prime contributor to environmental contamination. The Ciba-Geigy plant in Toms River, New Jersey, provides an example. It is situated on the banks of the Toms River just a few miles upstream from the mouth of the river on the Atlantic shore. The plant is one of the more attractive plants in the nation. It is located in a wooded suburban area, and Ciba-Geigy has gone out of its way to maintain a landscaped parkland setting. Unfortunately, conditions beneath the surface of the ground are not so pristine. A cocktail of organic chemicals including trichloroethylene and chlorobenzene defines a plume that

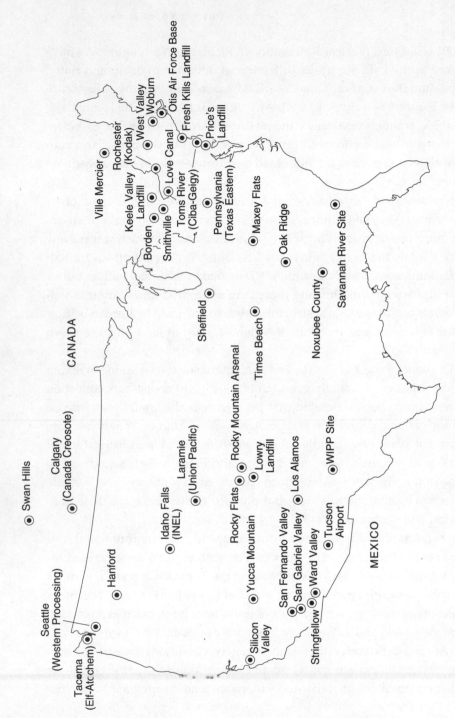

Figure 6. Contaminated sites and waste-management facilities mentioned in the text.

originates at the plant site and has historically discharged into the Toms River. In an ironic twist of fate, its path takes it directly beneath a subdivision that attracted home buyers by promising a well in every backyard. Many of these wells became contaminated and are now closed. Ciba-Geigy has instituted an expensive remedial program to prevent the discharge of chemicals into the river. In fact, the program is so expensive that it is rumored that the plant no longer generates any revenues to the company, but is kept in operation for the sole purpose of paying for its own environmental cleanup.

On the other side of the continent, on the shores of Commencement Bay near Tacoma, Washington, Elf-Atochem operates a chemical plant on a site that formerly manufactured the herbicide penite. This herbicide is an arsenic-based compound, and the site has been identified as a source of arsenic contamination in the bottom sediments of the Hylebos Waterway, which leads into Commencement Bay. The primary route of contaminant delivery is the discharge of arsenic-laden groundwater seepage into the waterway along its banks where it borders the plant boundary.

Every site is different, and the Elf-Atochem site has an interesting twist as well.[33] It turns out that the former operations also involved the disposal of waste brines into the sandy soils that blanket the site. These brines were sufficiently caustic that they dissolved large amounts of silica from the sand as they flowed through it. Then, when the brines discharged into the seawater in the Hylebos Waterway, a mixing reaction took place that precipitated out crystalline silica and plastered it onto the side of the bank as a thin, hard coating, just like the tufas one sees around the fumaroles in Yellowstone Park. This peculiar and unexpected chemical reaction has created a self-sealing process at the site that helps reduce the rate of discharge of the arsenic-contaminated groundwater into the waterway.

It would make a better story if I could stop here, but alas, technical studies at the site have indicated that this natural protection is not sufficient, so Elf-Atochem has also installed more traditional remedial measures in the form of a sheet-pile wall along the bank of the waterway and a pump-and-treat system on-site. Whatever benefits the silica may have provided on the shoreline are lost on the remediation engineers; the silica likes to precipitate in the treatment facility just as much as it does on the shoreline, fouling the equipment and confounding the arsenic removal from the contaminated groundwater.

Wood-treatment facilities have historically lacked proper environmental controls. Railroad ties and telephone poles were traditionally treated by immersing them in dip tanks of wood-preserving chemicals such as creosote and pentachlorophenol, and there has always been much attendant spillage and leakage of these chemicals.

The largest contaminated wood-preserving site in the nation is the Union Pacific Railroad site at Laramie, Wyoming. The Laramie Tie Plant site operated for almost 100 years, between 1886 and 1983, and these operations resulted in contamination of more than 100 acres at the site. When remedial activities began in 1983, there were almost 10 million gallons of wood-preserving liquids in the soils at the site, representing an average loss of *100,000 gallons per year* over the century of operations. That's 275 gallons of chemicals that mysteriously disappeared and had to be replaced each and every day! Luckily, contamination was concentrated in a thin, surficial sand layer that is underlain at shallow depth by a clay impermeable to the passage of the dense, viscous, wood-preserving liquids. Remedial actions have included rerouting the Laramie River away from the site, construction of a dike along the river to protect the site from flooding, and installation of a subsurface cutoff wall through the surficial sand to the underlying clay layer all around the contaminated area. This cutoff wall was constructed by trenching through the sand and then filling the trench with a low-permeability clay slurry. With a total length of almost two miles, it is probably the longest cutoff wall in the country (but far from the deepest). Thus contained, the site sits there in limbo. Driving by it, you would never know anything was amiss. There are currently no known technologies that could remove all the wood-preserving liquids, but as a kind of penance Union Pacific Railroad has made the site available to researchers who are trying to develop such techniques.

Another wood-preserving site, the Canada Creosote site in Calgary, Alberta, hit the news in the late eighties. This site, which sits on the banks of the Bow River, had been abandoned since 1962, covered over and filled in, and is now the site of two large car dealerships and a freeway interchange. In the late eighties, large blobs of creosote began to appear in the Bow River, a highly protected and pristine trout fishing stream. Eventually the blobs were traced back to the long-forgotten Canada Creosote site, and careful investigation there revealed the presence of more than 2 million gallons of creosote in a subsurface "pool" beneath the car dealerships. A cutoff wall has been constructed along the riverbank and a nervous watch is now under way to see whether the blobs will reappear.

The most ubiquitous of all the environmental contaminants are the solvents, and among the heaviest solvent users are the plants, contractors, and service companies of the aerospace industry. As a result, some of the best hunting ground for major solvent releases are in the vicinity of airports and military bases. The military-industrial complex is not dead; it's just out there polluting the environment.

In Tucson, Arizona, a solvent plume several hundred feet wide and more than five miles long has contaminated groundwater in the vicinity of the Tucson airport. The primary source area is thought to be the large Hughes Aircraft facility, but there are many other smaller plants and aerospace contractors in the vicinity who are also potential contributors.

In the San Fernando Valley near Los Angeles, California, just over the hills from the famous Hollywood sign, a large plume of solvent-contaminated groundwater emanates from the area around the Burbank airport. The primary source has been traced to one of the many facilities of the Lockheed Corporation in the area, but there are literally hundreds of smaller aerospace service companies nearby, and many of them have had documented solvent spills and leaks on their property. The contamination of the groundwater in the San Fernando Valley is particularly unfortunate because all the domestic water supplies for the 1 million people who live in the valley come from groundwater development. There is now a need for close integration of water-supply and water-contamination management in the basin that is stretching the administrative abilities of the responsible agencies. The water supply issues are administered by a watermaster, whose office must oversee the performance of thousands of wells and hundreds of water purveyors, with many complex water-trade agreements in place, and many past adjudications and court settlements to take into account. The water contamination issues fall under the Superfund program administered by the EPA. The agency has to deal with many potentially responsible parties, a complex cost recovery process, the ever present threat of litigation, and a situation where the optimal remedial action is unclear. Only time will tell whether the messy negotiations between these many parties, all with their own agendas and their own lawyers, will ever arrive at solutions that are technically and economically feasible.

I have already discussed some of the problems at the Hanford Nuclear Reservation in eastern Washington State, but Hanford is certainly not the only environmental legacy of the Manhattan Project. The Department of Energy (DOE), which now runs the nation's nuclear programs, has also been embarrassed by difficulties at its Rocky Flats site near Denver, Colorado. Rocky Flats is a weapons facility that first hit the news in 1969, when a serious fire there produced a large quantity of low-level, plutonium-contaminated debris (transuranic waste, in today's jargon). It was necessary to ship the waste in a hundred thousand sealed drums from Colorado to the Idaho National Engineering Laboratory near Idaho Falls, Idaho, where there were facilities available for its storage. This waste has been a political hot potato ever since. Its ultimate destination is supposed to be the Waste Isolation Pilot Plant (or WIPP site) near Carlsbad, New Mexico, but this underground repository for military nuclear waste, which is fully constructed and has been ready to receive waste for several years, has been prevented until very recently from going into operation by political and legal opposition.

Up until January 1992, the Rocky Flats plant was involved in manufacturing the plutonium component of nuclear weapons. It is a huge industrial site with hundreds of buildings spread over some four hundred acres. It sits in lonely isolation on its own little mesa, in the shadow of the Rockies and surrounded by the bald prairie. As with all large industrial sites, there is a long list of historical spills and leaks here, not just of radioactive material but also of more traditional contaminants like oils and solvents. In January 1992, the plant was closed, and the workforce (not all that much reduced in numbers) is now engaged solely in "environmental restoration, waste management, decontamination, and decommissioning." The name of the plant has been changed to the Rocky Flats Environmental Technology Site. We have our second example of a plant whose operation is totally dedicated to its own cleanup.

Much of the decommissioning effort at Rocky Flats revolves around security and control of the many surplus tons of weapons-grade plutonium still stored there. In December 1996, the DOE announced a twenty-year plan to dispose of the plutonium at a cost of $2.3 billion.[34] It will probably involve moving the plutonium either to the Hanford site or the Savannah River site near Aiken, South Carolina.

While the nation's high-level nuclear waste awaits the development of the repository at Yucca Mountain, Nevada, or the full use of the WIPP site in New Mexico, low-level waste from past programs has been stored at many sites across the nation.[35] Some are DOE facilities like those already mentioned at Hanford, Rocky Flats, Savannah River, and the Idaho National Engineering Laboratory, and those as yet unmentioned at Los Alamos, New Mexico, and Oak Ridge, Tennessee. Others are commercial operations, in such communities as Sheffield, Illinois; West Valley, New York; and Maxey Flats, Kentucky. These last three sites are now closed, two of them (West Valley and Maxey Flats) following charges of radioactive environmental contamination.

So what should we make of this roll call of infamy? My purpose is simply to show that major cases of environmental contamination are endemic across the nation (and indeed across all the developed nations of the world). They are largely a legacy of our past sins, but even our current technologies are not going to prevent similar occurrences in the future. Environmental policies ought to be based on a realistic appraisal of what we can and can't do about this situation.

THE BOTTOM LINE

- Waste is an unavoidable by-product of human life. There are waste streams generated at every stage in the product cycles that bring us the goods that make life enjoyable, and at every stage in the fuel cycles that provide the energy to drive our material way of life.

• Comparisons of alternative energy sources ought to take into account the benefits, costs, and risks across the entire fuel cycle of each alternative. Nuclear power represents a truly remarkable energy opportunity, but there is no denying that it involves risks that are different in kind from other energy sources. Given the growing energy needs of the world, it is unlikely that any of the feasible technologies will be abandoned. It is likely that environmental policies will have to continue to consider a mix of energy sources and the potential environmental consequences of all their respective fuel cycles.

• Hazardous waste containing toxic organic chemicals, metals, and radionuclides is generated at a rate on the order of 250 million tons per year. Almost all of it is industrial, much of it is liquid, and the rates of generation are more likely to increase than to decline.

• The safety factors used by engineers in the design of hazardous-waste landfills do not guarantee environmental protection, even in the short term. There are small but finite probabilities of failure associated with any engineering design.

• Landfills cannot last forever, even when multiple-barrier designs are claimed. The canisters, liners, and leachate collection systems that provide waste containment have a finite maximum life. Current design practices in the waste-management industry postpone failure of the engineered systems for tens to hundreds of years, but they do not prevent long-term contaminant releases to the environment.

• Contaminant releases to the environment also arise from accidents, spills, and leaks during the operation of industrial plants. Most such events can be traced to human error. Even very small spills, which are probably unavoidable in the course of normal industrial operations, can have a large environmental impact.

• Under the influence of discounting, the economic time horizon of the corporate owners of industrial plants and waste-management facilities is not likely to exceed 50 years. From their perspective, economic events that might happen after this time, including the possibility of regulatory penalties or the cost of site cleanup, are of no consequence to the decision-making process associated with initial facility design.

• Given the broad societal consensus that intergenerational environmental protection is in the public interest, then it is necessary for government to set regulatory environmental policies that will drive facility owners to seek designs that feature more long-lived environmental protection.

- Major cases of environmental contamination are endemic across the nation. Environmental policies should be based on a realistic appraisal of what we can and can't do about them.

3 Environmental Contamination

WHAT MATTERS AND WHAT DOESN'T

What matters and what doesn't? It sounds like a simple issue. Surely there can be no waffling on this one. Just give us the straight goods.

Well, as you may suspect, it is not to be. When it comes to assessing the impact of chemicals on human health, one has to peel the layers away carefully. We are at the intersection of science, medicine, politics, and law, with a strong flourish of human emotion thrown in to tangle the knot. The answers do not come easily.

In the first place, much less is known than you probably thought. Only a small percentage of the sixty-five thousand or so chemicals known to be in commercial use have been adequately tested for their effects on human health.[1] Second, there is far less consensus than you may have thought, even among reputable scientists. Results are controversial and interpretations differ.

There are actually two issues that must be addressed and they are separable. First, we want to identify those chemicals known to be harmful to human health under acute exposures (where an acute exposure is defined as one that takes place at a high dose over a short period of time). And second, for the chemicals so identified, we want to know whether the chronic exposures that will be experienced from environmental contamination are also likely to impact human health (where a chronic exposure is defined as one that takes place at a low dose over a long period of time). For any given chemical, assessment of the first issue requires the development of a toxicological profile, while assessment of the second issue requires a consideration of the dose-response relationship. The first of these topics is covered in the next section, and the second in a later section.

RATIONAL FEARS: TOXIC CHEMICALS, CANCER, GENETICS, AND FERTILITY

There are five types of studies that can be brought to bear on the question of whether a given chemical is harmful to human health: (1) studies of the impacts on individuals of acute accidental exposures, (2) occupational health studies on groups of workers in the chemical industry who have experienced larger exposures than the general population, (3) forensic studies designed to uncover correlations, or better yet, cause-effect relationships, for documented cases of health degradation, (4) public health studies that compare health impacts on exposed populations with those of unexposed control groups, and (5) laboratory animal studies that attempt to extrapolate the impacts of large doses imparted over a short time span to small animals (mice, rats, hamsters, and rabbits) to those that would be experienced from small doses imparted over a much longer time span to much larger animals (human beings).

The first four of these approaches can be grouped under the heading of epidemiological studies, in that they deal directly with human beings. Acute individual exposures often provide the best evidence of direct toxic impact. Occupational health studies long ago proved their worth when they identified the prevalence of silicosis in coal miners and lung cancer in asbestos workers. Forensic studies clarified the role of chemical exposures at Love Canal and Times Beach and in the Japanese rice-oil incident. Public health studies have, among their many contributions, confirmed the value of fluoridation of water supplies in the prevention of dental caries.

Unfortunately, epidemiological evidence is quite limited, both in terms of the number of chemicals for which data exists and in the number of studies available for those chemicals for which data does exist. For most chemicals we must turn to the animal data, which is available in abundance, and which is usually quite clear with respect to the animals tested. However, the defensibility of extrapolating these findings to human beings is not at all clear, and there is no consensus on the validity of this approach, either within the scientific community or outside of it.[2]

The health impacts that have been observed on animals or people from *acute* exposures to chemicals run the gruesome gamut from skin rashes and eye irritations to cancer and instant death. The impacts can be classified as: toxic, neurotoxic, carcinogenic, teratogenic, or mutagenic. Toxic effects can include nausea, blurred vision, numbness, skin rashes, headaches, and respiratory problems, as well as more serious damage to the internal organs such as the liver and kidneys. Neurotoxic effects impact the central nervous system, sometimes producing brain damage that can lead to depression, reduced learning capacity, and permanent neurological deficit. Carcinogenic impacts include leukemia, skin cancer, and cancer of the lungs, liver, kidneys, and stomach. Teratogenic impacts affect the reproductive system, leading to possible loss of fertility, damage to embryo and fetus, birth defects, miscarriage, and perinatal deaths (death of mother or child within a few months of birth). Mutagenic impacts attack the DNA in the cells of the body and lead to genetic diseases that are passed on to future generations.

Some of these impacts are targeted on specific organs (for example, the heavy metal cadmium attacks the kidneys); some are more systemic (radioactive exposure, for example). Some are immediate (cyanide poisoning); some are delayed (cancer). Some are irreversible (brain damage); some are reversible (liver damage). It is a scary list of possibilities that can lead to human tragedy, and anyone who tries to suggest that we can just forget about the evidence of acute exposures when thinking about chronic environmental exposures is not likely to receive a very responsive hearing from most of us.

It would be impossible to try to list every conceivable impact of every conceivable chemical. Instead, Table 3 presents a representative sampling of some of the more common toxic chemicals and a measure of their acute toxicological impact.[3] They are grouped as follows: (1) metals, with lead and arsenic leading the way; (2) petroleum hydrocarbons, the so-called BTEX components of oil and gasoline (for benzene, toluene, ethylene, and xylene), with benzene as the primary villain; (3) chlorinated organic solvents such as trichloroethylene, perchloroethylene, methylene chloride, chloroform, carbon tetrachloride, and the very bad actor, vinyl chloride; (4) wood preserving chemicals such as creosote and pentachlorophenol; (5) PCBs (for polychlorinated biphenyls), which I will discuss more fully in the next section; (6) dioxin, the most toxic chemical known; (7) pesticides, Rachel Carson's original nemesis; (8) radionuclides; and (9) bacteria and viruses.

The grouping in Table 3 is just for convenience; it is not a perfect chemical classification. Some of the listed chemicals are elements (like lead), some are ions (like the radionuclides), and some are compounds (like the solvents). Most of the compounds listed in Table 3 are specific individual chemicals, but a few represent sets of related chemicals with similar properties, like the chlorobenzenes, the PCBs, and the dioxins. One of the listings, creosote, is actually a mixture of many related chemicals, the so-called polycyclic aromatic hydrocarbons, the most common of which is naphthalene. Another of the listings is not a chemical at all: bacteria and viruses are living biological entities; they are listed in Table 3 so we won't forget about them.

Many of the chlorinated organic solvents and pesticides have long chemical names. To an organic chemist, this nomenclature has great significance. For example, a chemist knows, just from the name, that the chemical structure of trichloroethylene will be an ethylene chain with three attached chlorines (of course, this chemist also knows what an

Table 3 Toxicological profiles for selected chemicals.

Class	Contaminant	Acronym	Sources	Toxic	Neurotoxic	Carcinogenic	Teratogenic	Mutagenic
Metals	Lead		Batteries, paint, gas	#	#	E	#	
	Arsenic		Herbicides, glass	#		A	#	#
	Mercury		Paint, drugs	#	#	E	#	#
	Cadmium		Alloys			D	#	
	Chromium		Plating	#		D	#	#
Petroleum hydrocarbons	Benzene	BTEX	Solvents, drugs, oil, gasoline, dyes, textiles, explosives		#	A	#	#
	Toluene			#		D	#	
	Ethylene					E		
	Xylene			#	#	D	#	
	Hexachlorobenzene					B		
Chlorinated organic solvents	Trichloroethylene	TCE	Solvents	#	#	B	#	
	Perchloroethylene	PCE		#	#	B		
	Methylene chloride	MC		#	#	B		
	Chloroform			#	#	B		
	Carbon tetrachloride	CTC		#	#	B	#	
	Vinyl chloride	VC	Plastics	#	#	A	#	#

Category	Chemical	Abbreviation	Source		Class		
Wood preserving chemicals	Trichlorophenol		Wood preservatives	#	B	#	
	Pentachlorophenol	PCP		#	B	#	
	Creosote				B		
PCBs	Polychlorinated biphenyls	PCB	Insulators, transformers, pipelines	#	B	#	#
Dioxin	Dioxins		Incinerators	#	B	#	
Pesticides		DDT	Herbicides, fungicides, insecticides	#	B	#	#
		EDB			B	#	
	Chlordane			#	B		
	Toxaphene			#	B	#	
	Heptachlor				B		
	Lindane				B		
Radionuclides			Weapons facilities		A	#	
Bacteria and viruses			Poor sanitation	#			

ethylene chain is). For most of us, it will be handier to use the common acronyms presented in Table 3, for those chemicals that have acronyms: TCE (for trichloroethylene), PCB (for the polychlorinated biphenyls), DDT (for dichloro-diphenyl-trichloroethane), and so on. Some of these have become so common (like DDT) that the full names are seldom used, even by chemists. Some of these long generic names have not been listed in Table 3. The pesticide trade names, like heptachlor and toxaphene, also hide long generic names that have not been listed.

It is worth noting that while many of the chemicals listed in Table 3 are synthetic, not all of them are. Certainly, the heavy metals are naturally occurring, as are the radionuclides. The polycyclic aromatic hydrocarbons mentioned above occur naturally in crude oils. The popular environmentalist vision of humankind as the sorcerer's apprentice, totally responsible for placing a chemical curse on society, is not entirely accurate. There are natural hazards and synthetic hazards, and both deserve our attention.

The ubiquitous presence of chlorine in the organic compounds listed in Table 3 should not be overlooked. The fact that chlorine gas was used as a weapon in World War I is not surprising, nor is the fact that it did so much permanent damage to so many young men. Chlorinated organic chemicals (or more generally, halogenated organic chemicals, which may feature bromine or iodine in place of the chlorine) figure prominently in the toxicology of most animals, including human beings.

In the carcinogenic column of Table 3, the letters A through E refer to the EPA Carcinogen Classification System.[4] The classes are defined as follows: (A) *human carcinogens*, a classification given only to those chemicals for which there is sufficient epidemiological evidence to merit such a clear warning; (B) *probable human carcinogens*, for chemicals with sufficient evidence from animal studies, but limited or inadequate evidence from epidemiological studies; (C) *possible human carcinogens*, for chemicals with limited evidence from animal studies, and inadequate evidence from epidemiological studies; (D) *not classifiable*, due to lack of data; and (E) *noncarcinogenic to humans*, determined on the basis of adequate animal and/or epidemiological evidence. In these definitions, the adjective *sufficient* implies that there is evidence of tumors, either malignant or benign, in multiple experiments, multiple species, or to an unusual degree in one experiment or one species. The adjective *limited* implies that a cause-effect interpretation relating the chemical to cancer is credible, but that alternative explanations such as chance or bias cannot be excluded.

Only a few thousand chemicals have been fully tested, but these few thousand are among those thought most likely to be carcinogenic. Of these, only a few tens have been identified as certain human carcinogens. Several hundred have been tagged as possible or probable human carcinogens. However, not all these carcinogenic chemicals are equally potent. In fact, there may be as much as a millionfold difference in potency between the least potent carcinogen identified (saccharine) and the most potent (dioxin).[5] There is a general feeling among objective observers that any increase in societal cancer risk that can be ascribed to chemicals (and remember from chapter 1 that this total is only a few percent at most) will come from the proven human carcinogens in category A. The probable and possible human carcinogens could have a small influence on cancer risk, but it is likely to be below the threshold of current methods of forensic detection.[6]

When viewing Table 3 we must not let fear of cancer blind us to the importance of noncarcinogenic toxic effects. To those who suffer the consequences, there is nothing inconsequential about damage to liver and kidneys or the psychological trauma of a permanent neurological deficit. The ubiquitous solvent TCE, for example, is classified by the EPA as a "probable" carcinogen, implying some doubt (a doubt that seems appropriate, given the willingness of credible experts to testify on both sides of the issue at the leukemia trial in Woburn, Massachusetts),[7] but other health impacts are well documented. It is one of the few chemicals with a long-term study available that tracks the development of a permanent neurological deficit in an individual worker who experienced a single acute exposure.[8]

The risk of acute exposure to many of the chemicals in Table 3 has been much reduced over the years. The pesticide DDT has been essentially removed from our lives in response to the pleas of *Silent Spring*. PCB use in the United States has been phased out following passage of the Toxic Substances Control Act in 1976. Production of the solvent TCE is now less than a third of what it was in 1970 (but still totals more than 150 million pounds per year).[9] Of course, the affected industries have had to find alternative pesticides, lubricants, and solvents, and it is not really known whether the total health risk to humankind has been reduced or just the risk due to these specific chemicals.

One case where health benefits have certainly been realized is that of lead. Acute lead poisoning can do demonstrable harm, especially to children, as a result of inhalation of leaded gasoline fumes and contact with lead-based paints. Toxic effects take the form of seizures, comas, personality changes, and mental retardation. With mandated reductions in the use of lead-based paints and leaded gasoline, the amount of environmental lead carried in our bodies is also lessening. As noted by H. W. Lewis in his book *Technological Risk*, ''The control of lead poisoning is one of the success stories for environmental management. The threat was real and necessary measures were taken. Though the costs were high, they are a reasonable match to the benefits.''[10]

With all this talk of multisyllable organic contaminants and probable carcinogenic potency, there is a tendency to forget about good old-fashioned sanitation. Despite the almost universal presence of water treatment plants across the nation, public water supplies still occasionally fall out of compliance with respect to disease-carrying bacteria and viruses such as salmonella and cryptosporidium. The U.S. Centers for Disease Control and Prevention have monitored more than 600 major outbreaks of waterborne diseases since 1971.[11] The worst case occurred in Milwaukee, Wisconsin, in March 1993, where a cryptosporidium event affected more than 400,000 people, and 104 deaths were ascribed to the outbreak. If this latter figure is correct, and there is no reason to doubt it, it implies that considerably more immediate deaths are imposed on the nation from failure to control bacteria and viruses than have ever been ascribed to hazardous chemicals. (In fairness, it must be noted that it is difficult to compare the immediate individual deaths caused by viral epidemics with the cumulative carcinogenic effects and reduced longevity caused by chemical exposures. And if the comparison is made international, with the tragic releases from the chemical plant in Bhopal, India, included, the point is lost.)

Radionuclides represent a special class of carcinogens. Certain isotopes of certain elements (among them uranium, plutonium, radium, cesium, and iodine) are radioactive; that is, they spontaneously emit subatomic particles and electromagnetic radiation. It is now established beyond doubt that these radioactive emissions can cause cancer in living tissue. The environmental issues that arise from radioactive contamination are sufficiently different from those arising from chemical carcinogenesis that I will postpone further discussion of them until later in the book.

Table 3 is just a sampling of the chemicals that have been identified as toxic, carcinogenic, teratogenic, or mutagenic. The EPA's Priority Pollutants List, reproduced in Table 4, provides a longer list of suspected potential contaminants.[12] The grouping on the EPA list is in terms of the method of chemical analysis (base-neutral extractables, acid extractables, volatiles, pesticides, and inorganics). (One can only guess why the PCBs, which are not pesticides, are listed under the pesticides.) While the list is longer, most of the items on it fit into one of the nine groups in Table 3. For more detailed toxicological information on any particular chemical, the reader is directed to one of the many handbooks that provide summaries of individual toxicological profiles.[13]

So, if we return to the question posed in the title of this chapter (What matters and what doesn't?), we now have a partial answer in the form of a list of candidate chemicals that really matter. Over the years a semblance of consensus has arisen over which chemicals belong on the list and which don't. It's when we come to the questions of *how much* they matter and which ones *really, really* matter that the hackles are raised.

THE CONTROVERSY OVER THE HEALTH IMPACTS OF ORGANIC CHEMICALS: THE PCB STORY

In 1990, readers of the book *When Technology Wounds* would have learned that "one PCB molecule may be enough to damage your health, potentially causing vomiting, fatigue, the skin disease chloracne, liver damage, or cancer."[14] A reputable science news magazine carried the news that

Table 4 The EPA's Priority Pollutants List.

Base-Neutral Extractables

Acenaphthene	4-Chlorophenyl phenyl ether	Hexachlorobenzene
Acenaphthylene	Chrysene	Hexachlorobutadiene
Anthracene	Dibenzo[a,b]anthracene	Hexachlorocyclopentadiene
Benzidene	Di-n-butyl phthalate	Hexachloroethane
Benzo[a]anthracene	1,2-Dichlorobenzene	Indeno[1,2,3-cd] pyrene
Benzo[b]fluoranthene	1,3-Dichlorobenzene	Isophorone
Benzo[k]fluoranthene	1,4-Dichlorobenzene	Naphthalene
Benzo[ghi]perylene	3,3-Dichlorobenzidene	Nitrobenzene
Benzo[a]pyrene	Diethyl phthalate	N-Nitrosodimethylamine
Bis(2-chloroethoxy)methane	Dimethyl phthalate	N-Nitrosodiphenylamine
Bis(2-chloroethyl) ether	2,4-Dinitrotoluene	N-Nitrosodi-n-propylamine
Bis(2-chloroisopropyl) ether	2,6-Dinitrotoluene	Phenanthrene
Bis(2-ethylhexyl) phthalate	Di-n-octyl phthalate	Pyrene
4-Bromophenyl phenyl ether	1,2-Diphenylhydrazine	2,3,7,8-Tetrachlorodibenzo-p-dioxin
Butyl benzyl phthalate	Fluoranthene	1,2,4-Trichlorobenzene
2-Chloronaphthalene	Fluorene	

Acid Extractables

p-Chloro-m-cresol	4,6-Dinitro-o-cresol	Pentachlorophenol
2-Chlorophenol	2,4-Dinitrophenol	Phenol

2,4-Dichlorophenol	2-Nitrophenol	2,4,6-Trichlorophenol
2,4-Dimethylphenol	4-Nitrophenol	Total phenols

Volatiles

Acrolein	Chloroform	Ethylbenzene
Acrylonitrile	Chloromethane	Methylene chloride
Benzene	Dibromochloromethane	1,1,2,2-Tetrachloroethane
Bis(chloromethyl) ether	Dichlorofluoromethane	1,1,2,2-Tetrachloroethene
Bromodichloromethane	1,1-Dichloroethane	Toluene
Bromoform	1,2-Dichloroethane	1,1,1-Trichloroethane
Bromomethane	1,1-Dichloroethylene	1,1,2-Trichloroethane
Carbon tetrachloride	trans-1,2-Dichloroethylene	Trichloroethylene
Chlorobenzene	1,2-Dichloropropane	Trichlorofluoromethane
Chloroethane	cis-1,3-Dichloropropene	Vinyl chloride
2-Chloroethyl vinyl ether	trans-1,3-Dichloropropene	

Pesticides

Aldrin	Dieldren	PCB-1016*
alpha-BHC	alpha-Endosulfan	PCB-1221*
beta-BHC	beta-Endosulfan	PCB-1232*
gamma-BHC	Endosulfan sulfate	PCB-1242*
delta-BHC	Endrin	PCB-1248*
Chlordane	Endrin aldehyde	PCB-1254*
4,4'-DDD	Heptachlor	PCB-1260*
4,4'-DDE	Heptachlor epoxide	
4,4'-DDT	Toxaphene	

Table 4 *(continued)*

Inorganics

Antimony	Chromium	Nickel
Arsenic	Copper	Selenium
Asbestos	Cyanide	Silver
Beryllium	Lead	Thallium
Cadmium	Mercury	Zinc

*Not pesticides.

"PCBs are believed to cause cancer, still births, bone and joint deformities, skin rashes, and liver damage."[15] In congressional hearings in 1987, a U.S. senator stated that "PCB has been found to cause cancer and other illnesses."[16]

What then do we make of the statement by a reputable scientific author in 1993 that there is "no evidence that PCBs cause cancer in humans ... [n]or of any substantial adverse effect on human health from PCB exposure in the U.S."?[17] Or this statement from a reputable panel of toxicologists in 1989: "The panel concludes that the body of epidemiological evidence does not demonstrate any causal relationship between PCB exposure and any form of cancer"?[18]

What is going on here?

Well, what is going on with PCBs (and it is still going on) is a microcosm of the toxicological battles being fought over many toxic chemicals. At issue is the level of threat represented by *chronic* environmental exposures to chemicals known to be toxic on *acute* exposure.

If the PCB story were a play, it would have two distinct acts: the first act takes place in the period 1966–1976, leading up to the passage of the Toxic Substances Control Act (TSCA), and the second in the years since, which I am going to tell from the perspective of one of the unhappy players, the Texas Eastern Gas Pipeline Company.

In order to make sense of this story we first need to look past the initials, to the commercial and chemical properties that make PCBs special. From a commercial perspective, the property that sets PCBs apart is the fact that they are fire resistant. Starting with their introduction in the late 1920s through their phase-out after passage of the TSCA, they played an important industrial role as insulating materials, coolants, and lubricants. They were routinely used in the manufacture of plastics, adhesives, paint, newsprint, and fluorescent lights. Their most widespread use was as a nonflammable lubricant in electrical transformers. When they were first introduced, they were regarded as another synthetic miracle from the newly sanctified high priests of organic chemistry. They replaced flammable transformer lubricants, thus reducing the risk of fire in factories, offices, hospitals, and schools. Between 1929 and 1977, on the order of 1.2 billion pounds of PCBs were produced in the United States.[19]

From a chemical perspective, a *polychlorinated biphenyl* has an atomic structure described by its name. Like all organic chemicals, the basic building blocks are hydrogen and carbon. In a PCB, the hydrogen and carbon atoms are arranged in two phenyl rings (the *bi-phenyl* part), and one or more chlorine atoms (the *poly-chlorinated* part) attach themselves to the phenyl rings, as shown in Figure 7. There are 10 places for a single chlorine atom to attach itself, 24 ways for three chlorine atoms to distribute themselves, 46 ways for five chlorines, and so on. All in all, there are 209 possible atomic structures. Each of these atomic structures represents a different chemical compound. They are all PCBs, and they are all similar to be sure, but they are different nevertheless. In PCB parlance, they are known as *congeners*. Each congener has its own boiling point, its own solubility, and its own toxicological profile. In general, PCBs become more toxic as the number of chlorines in the atomic structure increases. Those few congeners with five or six chlorine atoms are far more toxic than the many congeners with only two or three.

To make matters more complicated, Monsanto, the sole domestic supplier of PCBs over their entire life span, chose to market them as mixtures of congeners rather than in their individual pure form. They used the trade name Aroclor, followed by a number, to identify the various mixes. The last two digits of the number reflect the percentage of chlorine in the mix. Aroclor 1242, 1254, and 1260 have 42 percent, 54 percent, and 60 percent chlorine respectively. From a toxicological perspective, Aroclor 1260 is a more potent contaminant than Aroclor 1242 because it contains considerably more chlorine.

And so to Act One. There are three scenes. In the first scene, in 1966, Swedish researchers report that unlike most organic chemicals, the biodegradation of PCBs in the environment occurs at a rate slower than the rate of acquisition, leading to the buildup of these compounds in soils around the world. Because of their low solubility in water and their affinity for adsorption on soils, they tend to be relatively immobile and to remain at the points of accumulation for many years. In the second scene, in 1968, the Japanese rice-oil incident occurs, with the blame traced to PCB contamination of the oils. More than 1,600 people are affected. Health impacts include severe skin lesions, liver damage, birth defects,

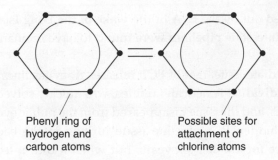

Phenyl ring of   Possible sites for
hydrogen and   attachment of
carbon atoms   chlorine atoms

Figure 7.   Chemical structure of PCBs.

and neurological disorders. In subsequent years, 51 deaths are ascribed to the incident. In the third scene, a set of well-documented studies carried out by the Centers for Disease Control in 1975 indicate that the ingestion of Aroclor 1260 causes liver cancer in rats.

The timing of these latter findings couldn't have been more propitious. It pushed the then ongoing hearings on the Toxic Substances Control Act into the public eye. A *New York Times* story identified PCBs as "cancer-causing agents" and one congressman was quoted as saying that the banning of PCBs was "a moral responsibility to the people."[20] As a result, Congress chose PCBs as the paradigm of all toxic substances, and it is the only chemical specified by name in the TSCA. There is no doubt about the intent of the TSCA; it banned the manufacture, processing, distribution, and use of all PCBs in all products (except those few in which the PCBs are "totally enclosed").

Act Two of the PCB story begins in January 1981, five years after passage of the TSCA, with PCBs presumably now long out of use. The public was surprised to learn that PCBs had been detected in a residential gas meter in suburban Long Island. The home was serviced by a utility that received its gas via a pipeline from Texas that was owned and operated by Texas Eastern Gas Pipelines. It turns out that PCB-based lubricants were widely used at compressor stations in the natural-gas pipeline industry prior to the TSCA. Even after conversion of the pipelines to different lubricants, small globules of the PCB oils remained trapped in the nooks and crannies of the system. In an industry-wide survey carried out by the EPA in the wake of the Long Island incident, 12 out of 31 interstate pipelines were found to have remnant PCB oils in their lines.

The immediate issue, that of PCB releases from gas lines into the residences of individual American families, was quickly solved by the utility companies, and the issue disappeared from the public eye. There was, however, a hidden PCB-pipeline issue lurking in the background. It didn't surface for another six years, but when it did, it led to another PCB brouhaha. It turns out that the PCB lubricants that leaked into the pipelines were not entrained in the natural gas itself but rather in the so-called *pipeline liquids* that condense out of the gas and accumulate in the low points of the pipeline system. These pipeline liquids are detrimental to efficient pipeline operation, and they are routinely removed from the lines by sending a tight-fitting pluglike device known as a "pig" through the pipeline from one compressor station to the next along the pipeline. This is not a trivial exercise. Texas Eastern, for example, has more than ten thousand miles of pipeline in two major pipeline systems that traverse fourteen states. It supplies ninety local gas distribution companies who supply natural gas to 15 million homes and businesses. Texas Eastern has hundreds of compressor stations along its lines, and at many of these, PCB-laden pipeline liquids were regularly removed from the lines with the pigs. For many years prior to the TSCA, and even afterward, these waste liquids were disposed of in open pits on the compressor station property. The EPA became aware of these pits as early as 1985, but the issue did not hit the newspapers until 1987. When it did, public fears were fanned by the media and, on March 17, 1987, specifically addressed at hearings held in a U.S. Senate subcommittee, entitled "Disposal of PCB Contaminated Liquids by the Texas Eastern Gas Pipeline Company."[21] In the upshot, Texas Eastern was fined $15 million and was forced to carry out remedial investigations that have cost the company another $25 million.

Given the high profile, one might assume that these investigations would uncover some very nasty news. However, that is not really the case. By 1994, a summary of the investigations was available.[22] It showed that the company had 76 sites where pipeline liquids had been disposed of in pits. Of these, only 27 indicated PCB levels above regulatory standards, and only 5 of these exhibited offsite contamination. In all cases the offsite migration was very local, usually involving low levels of contamination in springs emanating from the sites. In all these cases, Texas Eastern installed small, inexpensive collection and treatment systems, but no active recovery systems have been deemed necessary at any of the sites. Health risk calculations suggest that risks are minimal, and no adverse health effects have ever been documented at any of the Texas Eastern compressor stations. The EPA and several state agencies have approved the closure of these contaminated sites without further remedial action.

So it would seem that we have had somewhat of a tempest in a teapot. Act Two has had a run of seventeen years since the original PCB detection in the residential gas meter. There has been a lot of press, a lot of public concern, U.S. Senate hearings, and a large fine. What there has not been is any apparent adverse health impact.

In the years following the passage of the TSCA, there were many developments in the understanding of the health effects of PCBs. Later animal studies confirmed that Aroclor 1260 causes cancer in rats, but they also showed that Aroclor 1242 and 1254 do not. Only about 12 percent of Monsanto's production was in the form of Aroclor 1260, so there may be many industrial applications caught in the TSCA ban that perhaps ought not to be. On another front, occupational health studies carried out under the auspices of the National Institute for Occupational Safety and Health (NIOSH) found PCB levels in the blood of electrical equipment maintenance workers to be higher than in the general population. However, there was no statistically significant increase in cancer rates, nor any observable relationship between the length of employment in PCB-exposed jobs and health degradation.[23]

In a recently released ToxFAQs sheet, the U.S. Public Health Service states that "repeated skin contact to PCBs in rabbits caused liver, kidney and skin damage," and a "single large exposure to skin caused death in rabbits," but admits that "it is not clear if these effects would happen to people at similar levels of exposure." On the basis of these animal studies, the agency concludes that "PCBs may reasonably be anticipated to be carcinogens," but notes further that "studies in workers do not provide enough information to know with any certainty if PCBs cause cancer in humans."[24]

Philip Abelson, an editor of the respected journal *Science*, has taken the EPA to task for not using updated information in its regulatory decision-making. In a 1991 editorial, he quotes favorably the position of a former EPA administrator: "The current cancer policy is clearly overstating the cancer risks associated with many exposures to PCBs in the environment. In a number of instances it is driving regulatory decisions that, by any standard are a major economic impact for, at best, trivial public health gain."[25] Both Abelson and the former administrator are particularly critical of the failure to differentiate between high-chlorine and low-chlorine congeners in the PCB regulations.

So, is this the bottom line? Well, not quite. In the last two or three years, two new issues have been put on the table. The first represents a new spin on the long-recognized fact that PCBs (along with dioxins and pesticides) tend to accumulate in the environment. These *persistent organic pollutants* (now with the catchy acronym POPs) are apparently capable of migrating through the atmosphere as gases and aerosols on a global scale. There is a tendency for such gases to be volatilized in high-temperature regions of the earth and condensed in low-temperature regions. This could lead to the global migration of PCBs from the tropics to the poles, with preferential accumulations in these cold environments. There is concern that, if confirmed by ongoing studies, this phenomenon could threaten arctic and antarctic environments.[26]

The second development is the widely reviewed publication of the book *Our Stolen Future*,[27] which is hailed in a preface by Vice-President Al Gore as a second *Silent Spring*. The book links prebirth exposure to persistent organic pollutants, including PCBs, to a wide suite of reproductive health problems including fetal brain damage and global reductions in male sperm counts (a phenomenon that the authors admit is disputed by many scientists). The latest battleground for testing the thesis of *Our Stolen Future* is a set of data that has been available for some years on the long-term health of a group of women (and their children) who were known to have consumed inordinate amounts of PCB-contaminated fish from Lake Michigan. Previous studies documented higher PCB blood levels in the women but failed to discern any associated health effects.[28] Recently, however, researchers at Wayne State University in Detroit claim to have identified the effects of fetal brain damage in the children. The effects are held to be comparable to those found in children exposed to environmental lead.[29]

On the PCB question, and similarly with respect to many other toxic chemicals, we continue to be buffeted back and forth by the experts. It is obvious from the acute toxicological profiles that there is reason for concern, and there are some scientists who continue to wave warning flags in our faces at regular intervals. On the other hand, many reputable scientists downplay the health risks that could accrue from environmental accumulations of these persistent organic pollutants. For the PCBs at least, it seems clear from the facts that precious little harm has ever been documented. At the end we are left with uncertainty, and this uncertainty is apparently irreducible with the current level of available data.

The manner in which we cope with this uncertainty will be controlled in large part by our attitude toward risk. The level of protection we demand will depend on our perceptions of the level of risk posed by environmental contamination, and on the degree to which we are averse to such risks. To make our way toward an exploration of these topics, we must first consider the concepts of contaminant dose and dose-response and look at how current regulatory frameworks try to protect us.

EXPOSURE, DOSE, AND DOSE-RESPONSE

We now return to one of the questions raised at the beginning of this chapter: the relation between acute and chronic exposure. First of all, there is no question that there is a difference between the acute occupational exposures suffered by workers in industrial accidents and the chronic environmental exposures experienced by the population at large due to the presence of contaminated sites. The former occur at high doses and usually for a single brief period. The latter occur at low doses (at least 1,000 times less in most cases) through repeated contact over long periods of time (perhaps even a lifetime).

Environmental exposure may take place in the form of direct dermal contact with contaminated soils, through inhalation of contaminated air, or through the ingestion of contaminated food or water. For our purposes, I will limit discussion to the ingestion of contaminated drinking water. The ideas are easily transferable to the other exposure pathways. I will further assume that the contaminated drinking water comes from a water supply system that taps groundwater from an aquifer that may be affected by contaminants from a waste-management facility or other land-based industrial source of contamination.

If there are contaminants in groundwater at a significant distance from the presumed source, the contaminants will be in dissolved form. The strength of the contamination is defined by the concentration of the suspect chemicals. Concentration is defined as the mass of chemical in a given volume of water. It is usually measured in the metric units milligrams per liter (mg/L). For dissolved contaminants that don't change the density of the water (and hardly any of them do), 1 mg/L is numerically equivalent to 1 part per million (ppm); that is, for every million gallons of water, there is one gallon of the contaminating chemical dissolved evenly throughout it.

For each chemical there is an upper limit to the amount that can dissolve in water. This value, the solubility of the chemical in water, is also measured in mg/L or ppm. The solubility of the solvent TCE, for example, is 1,100 mg/L.[30] Some of the other solvents, like methylene chloride, are more soluble, while others, like carbon tetrachloride, are less so. However, water from your tap, even if it were to come from a contaminated aquifer, would be unlikely to exhibit concentrations that approach the solubility limit. There are mixing processes in the aquifer that lead to dilution and reduce the concentrations of the ingested water, usually by at least an order of magnitude (a factor of ten), and sometimes much more. Measured concentrations of TCE in contaminated aquifers seldom exceed 10 mg/L and are often less than 1 mg/L.

The dose received by an individual through ingestion of contaminated water is defined as the number of milligrams of chemical ingested per kilogram of body weight per day (mg/kg/day). A 70-kg individual (154 pounds) who drinks 2 liters of water per day (about half a gallon) that is contaminated with TCE at 1 mg/L is receiving a dose of about 0.03 mg/kg/day.

Everything to this point is straightforward and noncontroversial. But now the going gets sticky. We are interested in the health impact of these ingested doses on human beings. What we would like to have is a dose-response relationship that would tell us what type of toxic, carcinogenic, mutagenic, or teratogenic response will be incurred by human beings exposed to each specific chemical of concern at the appropriate environmental dose levels. Unfortunately (or fortunately, actually), scientists are not allowed to experiment on human beings, so direct evidence is absent. There is little epidemiological data available for many chemicals, and that which is available is almost all for acute exposure. Nor are forensic studies much help; as we learned with respect to the Woburn case and the Texas Eastern PCB sites, forensic studies of exposed human populations at low doses have been rare, equivocal, and controversial.

Under the circumstances, toxicologists have little choice but to turn to animal experiments. The data from the animal experiments must then be extrapolated to human beings. It is a crude and flawed approach, and there is little scientific consensus on either the procedures or the validity of the results, but at this point in the development of the science of toxicology it is the only available systemic approach. There is of course much ongoing medical research into the causal mechanisms that lead to kidney damage, or attacks on the central nervous system, or the initiation and promotion of cancer. Some day it may be possible to develop human dose-response relationships that are based on such mechanistic understanding of the impact of toxic chemicals on human organs, but such an approach is nowhere near possible today.

In animal experiments, small animals such as mice and rats are administered doses that are usually 100 to 10,000 times the environmental doses likely to be experienced by human receptors.[31] Some toxic endpoint must be specified as the response, and this endpoint is then plotted against the dose, as shown in Figure 8a. Any easily identified endpoint may be specified but the most common endpoint is death. In Figure 8

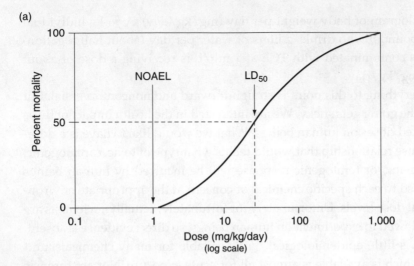

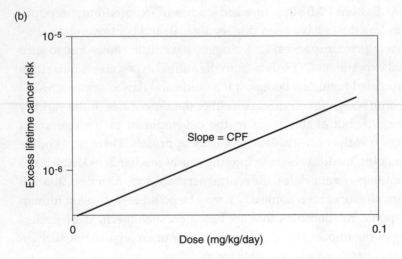

Figure 8. Dose-response relationships for (a) noncarcinogenic and (b) carcinogenic chemicals.

(which is a purely hypothetical example for the purposes of illustration), as the dose increases by factors of ten, the death rate of the experimental animal population also increases. The dose labeled LD_{50} is known as the median lethal dose. It is the dose in mg/kg/day at which only 50 percent of the animals survive the chemical assault. One can gain an indication of the relative toxicity of different chemicals by comparing their LD_{50} values for a particular species of experimental animal. For example, a sampling of the *single-exposure* oral LD_{50} values (measured in mg/kg rather than mg/kg/day) for the rat indicates values of 3,800 mg/kg for table salt, 115 mg/kg for DDT, 2 mg/kg for the pesticide parathion, and 0.02 mg/kg for dioxin.[32]

Animal experiments carried out over a very wide range in dose often exhibit a threshold dose below which there is no observable adverse effect of any kind in any of the test animals. This dose level is indicated as *NOAEL* in Figure 8a. The question arises as to whether a similar threshold can be anticipated in the human dose-response relationship, and if so, how one might extrapolate from the animal data to the human case. This issue is fraught with controversy. Current regulatory practice is to differentiate between noncarcinogenic and carcinogenic chemicals. For noncarcinogenic chemicals, consideration of a threshold is deemed acceptable, but for carcinogenic chemicals it is not.[33] Even for the non-carcinogens, the human NOAEL is calculated in a very conservative manner. It is taken as the animal NOAEL divided by a safety factor that depends on the animal used in the experiments, the chemical in question, and the assumed sensitivity of the human receptors. The safety factor usually falls in the range 100 to 1,000, meaning that human NOAELs are taken as two to three orders of magnitude less than animal NOAELs for the same chemical.[34]

If this degree of conservatism is not high enough for you, it turns out that there is yet another aspect of the methodology that adds a further layer of safety. For any given chemical, the line shown in Figure 8a is really a regression line drawn through a cloud of dots. Each dot would represent one animal experiment at a particular dose. Some of the dots would fall above the regression line and some below. In other words, the regression line represents the most likely estimate of the dose-response relationship, given the uncertainty indicated by the spread in the available experimental data. In some studies it has become the practice to use the 95th percentile regression line rather than the most likely regression line. This is the line drawn through the cloud of dots such that only 5 percent of the dots fall above the line and 95 percent fall below. When this line is extrapolated down to the horizontal coordinate line representing zero percent mortality, it leads to much smaller NOAEL values than would be obtained from a similar extrapolation of the most likely regression line. The argument made for its use is that it represents the dose-response for the most sensitive individuals in the exposed population.

For carcinogenic chemicals, the response is taken to be the number of excess cancers experienced by the exposed population as a result of the dose administered. Excess cancers are those that occur over and above the background cancer rate. At low doses (i.e., at doses well below those administered to animals in animal experiments), the human dose-response curve is assumed to be a linear relationship with no threshold, as shown in Figure 8b. The slope of this line defines the carcinogenic potency factor, or CPF. It is a measure of the potency of a given chemical as a cancer-causing agent. It is quoted in units of lifetime excess cancer risk per milligram (of contaminant) per kilogram (body weight) per day. The CPFs for various carcinogens can vary over many orders of magnitude. For example, the marginal probability of getting cancer that accrues to a 70-kg adult over a 70-year lifetime from drinking 2 L of water per day that is contaminated at a concentration of 0.1 mg/L is approximately 1 in 100,000 for TCE, 1 in 1,000 for vinyl chloride (VC), and 1 in 10 for the banned pesticide EDB.

For potentially carcinogenic chemicals, then, there are two issues that must be kept separately in mind: the likelihood that a chemical is a human carcinogen (indicated by its A, B, C, D, or E rating), and the potency of the chemical as a human carcinogen, if indeed it is one (indicated by its CPF).

There is a societal demand for regulatory agencies to put regulations in place such that no human receptor will receive an unacceptable dose from chronic environmental exposure to any chemical leading to an adverse carcinogenic or noncarcinogenic health impact. In most jurisdictions, one or both of two approaches have been encoded in the regulations. One approach makes use of legislated water quality standards, and the other relies on quantitative health-risk analysis. It will be instructive to look now at each of these approaches in turn.

RISK-BASED REGULATORY STANDARDS AND
THE ONE-IN-A-MILLION DECISION

The general idea of setting water quality standards as a guide to safe drinking water has a long history. Ever since the development of the first community water supply systems, it has been recognized that too much of a good thing can be a bad thing. Even the naturally occurring constituents that give water its pleasant thirst-quenching taste—sodium, calcium, magnesium, chloride, sulfate, and carbonate—have recommended maximum concentration limits above which the quality of the water is not considered acceptable for human consumption. In most cases the acceptability or unacceptability for these constituents is based on aesthetics rather than fear of serious toxic impact. Water with too much sodium chloride gets too salty to drink; water with too much sodium bicarbonate has a laxative effect on tourists. Mind you, some of the early limits *were* based on health concerns, as with bacterial counts, or on a general knowledge of the toxic properties of some constituents, like arsenic and cyanide. However, it was not until the environmental awakening of the sixties and seventies that people realized that health protection was needed from the myriad organic chemicals that had been allowed to contaminate streams and groundwater aquifers. With the formation of the Environmental Protection Agency in 1970, and settlement of the Natural Resources Defense Council suit that gave birth to the Priority Pollutants List in 1978, the stage was set for the next logical step: the setting of maximum contaminant levels for the priority pollutants. This was done under the auspices of the already established Safe Drinking Water Act.[35]

For noncarcinogenic toxic chemicals, the MCLs were set on the basis of the concept of an *acceptable daily intake* (ADI) for each chemical. The ADI is in turn based on the human NOAEL (the no observable adverse effect level introduced in the last section) for that chemical. Recall that the human NOAEL is calculated from the animal-based NOAEL using a very conservative set of safety factors. It has units of milligrams of contaminant per kilogram body weight per day. If it is assumed that the average human body weight is 70 kilograms (an average of adult male and female body weights), then for a human NOAEL of 0.001 mg/kg/day, the ADI of the chemical would be 0.07 mg/day. If it is further assumed that the average daily water intake for an individual is on the order of 2 liters/day, then the calculated MCL is 0.035 mg/L (i.e., 0.07 mg in 2 liters).

Most MCLs, especially those for organic chemicals, are well below 1 mg/L, so it has become common to specify them in units of micrograms per liter (μg/L), where a microgram is one-millionth of a gram, or one-thousandth of a milligram. The MCL of 0.035 mg/L calculated above would then be quoted at 35 μg/L. One μg/L is numerically equivalent to one part per billion (ppb).

For carcinogenic chemicals, a different approach was followed. It was desired to base the MCLs for these compounds on their carcinogenic potency factors, also introduced in the last section. Recall that this parameter also reflects a very conservative set of assumptions, including the no-threshold assumption and the use of a linear dose-response extrapolation from high to low doses. Recall also that the response in the dose-response relationship is in terms of the number of excess cancers experienced by the exposed population. In order to set an MCL, it was therefore necessary to select a value for the number of excess cancers resulting from the presence of environmental contamination, that would be considered acceptable in the population at large. In an in-house decision that has turned out to have far-reaching implications, the EPA selected the value of 1 in 1 million. It decided that the maximum contaminant levels for carcinogenic chemicals should be set such that the number of excess cancers due to environmental contamination will be less than 1 case in a population of 1 million people.

Once again, the 70-kg body weight and a water intake rate of 2 liters per day were assumed. Using the appropriate CPF for TCE (0.01 excess cancers/mg/kg/day), for example, together with the above assumptions and the 1-in-1-million goal, an MCL for TCE of 5 µg/L was established. It is worth noting that this value is three orders of magnitude below the range of commonly observed concentrations of TCE in contaminated aquifers (i.e., one-thousandth of these values), and almost six orders of magnitude below the TCE solubility limit (i.e., one-millionth of this value).

There was no particular justification for the 1 in 1 million decision that lead to this and other carcinogenic MCLs. It was simply a value that the EPA thought would be societally acceptable in the early risk-averse days of the environmental movement. The number can be traced to earlier deliberations at the Food and Drug Administration and the National Cancer Institute, but as one of the institute researchers of that era has been quoted saying, "We just pulled it out of a hat."[36]

Table 5 lists the established or proposed MCLs (in µg/L, or ppb) for the contaminants shown in Table 3.[37] They span nine orders of magnitude, from 0.00005 µg/L for dioxin to 10,000 µg/L for xylene. If the inordinately high and low values for these two chemicals are ignored, the rest of the values span slightly more than four orders of magnitude. The higher values imply that a chemical is less toxic; we need less protection from it. The lower values apply to the more toxic chemicals. No matter how you judge it, there is a great spread in the toxic potency of this suite of potential contaminants.

The primary purpose in establishing MCLs for toxic chemicals in water was to ensure safe drinking water for the population. However, the MCLs also play an important regulatory role at sites that fall under investigation in the Superfund program. Sites where groundwater concentrations are found to be above the MCLs for any of the priority pollutants are considered to be out of compliance with the regulations and are thus identified as contaminated sites requiring remedial action. This is the case even if the groundwater at the site is not connected to a drinking-water aquifer. There have been loud cries from the owners of such sites that the MCLs are too stringent for this purpose and their enforcement is driving expensive remedial actions at sites that do not represent a true threat to human health.

While one might question the motives of this constituency, there has

Table 5   Maximum contaminant levels (MCLs) for selected chemicals.

Class	Contaminant	MCL (µg/L)
Metals	Lead	15
	Arsenic	50
	Mercury	2
	Cadmium	5
	Chromium	100
Petroleum hydrocarbons	Benzene	5
	Toluene	1000
	Ethylene	—
	Xylene	10000
	Hexachlorobenzene	1
Chlorinated organic solvents	Trichloroethylene (TCE)	5
	Perchloroethylene (PCE)	5
	Methylene chloride (MC)	5
	Chloroform	—
	Carbon tetrachloride (CTC)	5
	Vinyl chloride (VC)	2
Wood-preserving chemicals	Trichlorophenol	—
	Pentachlorophenol (PCP)	1
	Creosote	—
PCBs	Polychlorinated biphenyls	0.5
Dioxins	Dioxins	0.00005
Pesticides	DDT	—
	EDB	0.05
	Chlordane	2
	Heptachlor	0.4
	Toxaphene	3
	Lindane	0.2

Source of data used in table: C. W. Fetter, *Contaminant Hydrogeology* (Englewood Cliffs, N.J.: Prentice Hall, 1993).

also been a growing consensus in the scientific community that the MCLs for many of the EPA priority pollutants are overconservative,[38] certainly with respect to their Superfund application, and perhaps even with respect to their direct application to drinking water. Critics raise several points: (1) the innate conservativeness of the 1 in 1 million framework, (2) the unwillingness to recognize the possible existence of threshold doses for carcinogenic chemicals, (3) the use of a linear dose-response relationship that leads to lower MCLs than the more defensible S-shaped curve, (4) the use of arbitrary safety factors of 100 and 1,000 in the extrapolation from animal to human dose-response relationships, and (5) the use of the 95th percentile dose-response relationship. Howard Holme, an environmental lawyer who has been particularly critical of EPA policy, has argued that most organic MCLs are at least 100 times too low, and could be raised by this factor without harm to human health.[39]

While the original federal MCLs were set within the 1 in 1 million framework, there has been a legislative trend in recent years, especially in state regulatory programs, to mandate even lower compliance limits. This legislative activity, which flies in the face of technical concerns to the contrary, usually occurs in response to public alarm engendered by specific local contaminant incidents that receive high-profile media coverage. The result is a tendency for ratcheting,[40] wherein periodic political pressures lead to more restrictive standards, but there is seldom any balancing pressure for relaxation. As noted by one critic of this practice, "Standards that were arbitrary in the first place are neither more or less arbitrary when tightened."[41]

There has also been a tendency to bring MCLs down as the technologies of analytical chemistry have improved.[42] At the same time that the EPA set the maximum contaminant levels (MCLs), it also set maximum contaminant level goals (MCLGs). For many of the most toxic organic chemicals (like dioxin and vinyl chloride) the MCLGs were set at zero. The reason that the MCLs did not match the MCLGs often lay in the inability of then-current analytical techniques to measure concentrations at the desired levels. There seemed little purpose in setting an MCL so low that it could not be measured. In recent years, however, there have been order-of-magnitude improvements in the detection limits for many organic chemicals. As the detection limits have come down from parts per million to parts per billion to parts per trillion (for some constituents), there has been a concomitant demand that MCLs be brought more into line with these new realities and with the original MCLGs.

In a thoughtful essay that I believe lays out a reasonable position, Robert Harris of Environ Corporation addressed the issue of whether the approaches currently used to set health protection goals are reasonable.[43] He concluded that the MCLs promulgated by the EPA are generally reasonable for deciding on the potability of public water supplies. They are very conservative but that is probably desirable in such situations. It must be remembered that the MCLs were promulgated under the Safe Drinking Water Act, and there is little doubt that the public demands absolute safety in this regard. The problems arise, in Harris's opinion, not from the MCLs themselves, but in their adoption for use in very different circumstances, in particular for the identification of contaminated sites and as the trigger for remedial action at such sites. Each of these sites is different, and they do not all threaten drinking-water supplies.

In these circumstances, one would like to turn to a methodology that provides a more site-specific assessment of actual health risks. Such methods of health risk assessment exist, and in principle their application makes a lot of sense; but alas, as we are about to see, there are problems here too in the current style of application.

DIRT-EATING DWARFS AND AGORAPHOBIC
BASEMENT DWELLERS: THE ARCANE WORLD
OF HEALTH RISK ANALYSIS

I have already introduced the concept of risk in chapter 2. The context there was in terms of an economic risk analysis carried out by the owner-operator of a landfill in the throes of making difficult and costly design decisions. The risk was defined there as the probability of failure of the landfill multiplied by the dollar consequences of such a failure to the owner-operator. We now turn to the concept of risk in the context of a health risk analysis. Once again, risk is defined as a probability times a consequence, but now our perspective is changed, from that of an owner-operator protecting his or her own economic interests, to that of a regulatory agency protecting societal interests. The unwanted consequences in this case are disease, reduced longevity, and death. The probability in this case is the probability of a human receptor receiving a dose sufficient to produce these consequences as a result of contaminants released to the environment at a contaminated site. For carcinogenic chemicals, a health risk analysis for a specific contaminated site produces a probability of exposure that can be compared with the acceptable risk of 1 in 1 million.

A quantitative health risk evaluation involves five steps, many of them closely related to the concepts introduced in the previous sections.[44] Step 1 is the selection of a few representative indicator chemicals or contaminants of concern from among those known to have been released at the contaminated site. The indicator chemicals ought to include both carcinogens and noncarcinogens (if both are present at the site), and they should include both the most common contaminants at the site and the most toxic.

Step 2 is the exposure assessment, in which the fate of the contaminant release is assessed, and the nature of the possible transport of the contaminants from the site to potential receptors is considered. In most cases, the primary threat occurs in offsite transport by groundwater flow, and the primary exposure pathway is the ingestion of water from a water supply system that taps a contaminated groundwater aquifer. The fate and transport of contaminants at a specific site are controlled in part by the properties of the chemicals—for example, their affinity for adsorption on soils, their solubility in water, and their potential to be biodegraded by microorganisms—and in part by the nature of the hydrogeological environment into which they are released, in particular the type of soils or rocks present at the site, and the direction and rate of groundwater flow. This is the step that the owner of a contaminated site hopes will get him or her off the hook. Even though contaminant MCLs may be exceeded in on-site monitoring wells, there is some possibility that the delivery of these contaminants to potential receptors will be sufficiently attenuated that no health risk is actually realized. A more complete discussion of source areas, groundwater plumes, and contaminant transport is included in chapter 4.

Step 3 involves the estimation of potential chemical intakes by the receptor population, whether by ingestion, inhalation, or dermal contact. For the ingestion of groundwater, the doses incurred are directly related to the concentrations of the contaminants in the water.

Step 4 is the toxicity assessment, which involves application of the acceptable daily intakes for noncarcinogenic chemicals and the carcinogenic potency factors for carcinogenic chemicals. For most common contaminants of concern, the recommended ADI and CPF values are available in published listings.[45]

Step 5 is the risk characterization. For carcinogenic risk from ingestion of contaminated groundwater, the excess lifetime cancer risk is calculated as the CPF (excess lifetime cancer risk/mg/kg/day) times the concentration of the chemical in the water (in mg/L) times the average daily intake of water (2 L/day) divided by the assumed body weight of a representative receptor (70 kg). If this risk is less than 1 in 1 million (10^{-6}), it is deemed to be an acceptable risk; if it is greater, it is unacceptable.

There is a growing recognition in many jurisdictions, including the EPA Superfund program, that forcing remedial action at contaminated sites solely on the basis of MCLs in monitoring wells at the site is leading to large remedial expenditures that are not necessary to protect human health. The health-risk-analysis approach, which is gaining popularity in this period of environmental reaction, provides a more direct estimate of the threat to human health from contaminated sites.

Or at least it does in principle. In reality, quantitative risk assessment is open to many of the same criticisms leveled at the methods used to develop the MCLs. The current risk assessment protocols also rely on the 1 in 1 million criteria, and they too depend on ADI and CPF values that may be orders of magnitude more conservative than necessary. In fact, the quantitative risk assessments introduce yet another layer of conservativeness into the mix. In Step 3, in the estimation of chemical intakes, regulatory agencies have developed a tendency to demand exposure scenarios that are so conservative that in some cases they become truly silly. In the first place, all receptors are often taken to be children, thus halving the pertinent body weights. In one typical example, a child receptor was assumed to eat two teaspoonfuls of contaminated dirt each and every day for several years.[46] In another, fumes from a volatile organic chemical dissolved in groundwater were assumed to leak into a basement room, there to be inhaled by a human receptor twenty-four hours a day for an entire 70-year lifetime. Some critics argue that these unrealistic scenarios, coupled with the conservative assumptions and safety factors inherent in the toxicity assessment, can lead to risk estimates that exceed the actual risk by as much as a millionfold.[47]

There are some counterarguments that can be made to these attacks on the current risk-analysis methodology.[48] There are cases in history where chemicals (for example, the drug thalidomide) that were not harmful to animals turned out to be very harmful to humans. There is also the question of whether complex chemical mixtures might have synergistic effects leading to greater toxicity than that ascribed to individual chemicals. Another issue is whether current methodologies adequately take into account bioaccumulations up the food chain (as may have affected the children of the women whose diet included the contaminated Lake Michigan fish). Lastly, there is the question of future receptors. When one is dealing with very long time horizons, on the order of hundreds or thousands of years, as, for example, in the design of nuclear waste repositories, the argument can be made that it is impossible to predict future population growth and demographic distributions. Who, for instance, in 1850, would ever have foreseen the birth and growth of Las Vegas and its sun-and-fun economy on the desert? As the saying goes, "Prediction is very easy, except into the future."

While these counterarguments have some merit, I believe that the degree to which they might lead to underestimation of health risks is overwhelmed by the many layers of conservativeness in the basic methodology. I cannot subscribe to the estimate of a millionfold, but I believe that the health risks from contaminated sites currently tend to be significantly overestimated, perhaps by as much as two orders of magnitude. There is a justifiable need for conservativeness when dealing with public health, but as we shall see in succeeding chapters, our averseness to risk is leading to massive societal expenditures that may not be doing us much good and might better be spent on other environmental or social ills.

RISK PERCEPTION, RISK AVERSION, AND ACCEPTABLE RISK

It is almost a parlor game among risk experts to make light of the public's risk perceptions. It is "flavored by emotion, steeped in biases, and limited by lack of education."[49] Why is it, they ask, that in these times, "when there is less risk than ever before, there is more concern than ever before?"[50] Commenting on the Alar apple scare, one expert noted that in most cases "the risk of consuming the apples is lower than the risk of driving to the store to buy them."[51]

There is no question that there are systemic differences between experts and laypeople in their perception of risk. Table 6 displays the results of a poll comparing responses from toxicologists and laypeople regarding the threat posed by carcinogenic chemicals.[52] The toxicologists are consistently more sanguine and the laypeople are consistently more concerned. In another study, members of the public ranked environmental chemicals (in particular, pesticides) among the top ten perceived risks facing humankind (out of ninety), along with nuclear weapons, war, and terrorism.[53] (In case you're interested, fluorescent lights, marijuana, and roller coasters all fell into the bottom ten.) Risk experts do not rank chemically based health risks nearly so high. For example, one toxicological review paper calculated that the risk of getting cancer from drinking one can of beer (as a result of its ethyl alcohol content) or one can of cola (as a result of its formaldehyde content) is far greater than the risk of getting cancer from drinking one liter of water from the most contaminated well in Silicon Valley (which contained 2,800 mg/L TCE).[54]

In this same study, the authors calculated that the risk of getting cancer from the contaminated Silicon Valley well water was only four times that of ordinary tap water. This surprising conclusion has more to do

Table 6   Results of a poll comparing responses between toxicologists and lay-people regarding carcinogenic chemicals.

Statement	Percent Toxicologists in Agreement	Percent Laypeople in Agreement
"There is no safe level of exposure to a cancer-causing agent."	19%	54%
"People are unnecessarily frightened about very small amounts of pesticides found in groundwater."	67%	24%
"A one-in-a-million lifetime risk of cancer from exposure to a particular chemical is too small a risk to worry about."	93%	59%

Source of data used in table: Robert S. Raucher, "The Economic Value of Groundwater Protection: What Are the Benefits and How Do They Compare to the Costs?" *GSA Today* 3 (July 1993): 183–94.

with the tap water than it does with the well water. Although they may not be aware of it, most people in North America are exposed to chlorinated chemicals every day in their tap water.[55] The water chlorination process that protects us against pathogenic diseases reacts with the naturally occurring organic constituents in water to form a class of chlorinated chemicals called trihalomethanes. These compounds are similar to (and in some cases, identical with) the chemicals found in contaminated groundwater. The average chlorinated tap water in the United States contains 83 μg/L chloroform, a chemical that appears in Table 4 as an EPA priority pollutant. There are situations in the United States where remedial actions at contaminated sites have been triggered by concentrations of chlorinated organic chemicals that are lower than those present in local tap water.

Table 7 provides a list of actions that increase the risk of death by 1 in 1 million: smoking one and a half cigarettes, drinking a half liter of wine, or driving thirty miles in a car.[56] This is the same risk used to

Table 7   Actions that increase the risk of death by one in a million.

Action
Smoking 1.4 cigarettes.
Drinking 0.5 liters of wine.
Spending 3 hours in a coal mine.
Traveling 30 miles by car.
Flying 1,000 miles by commercial jet.
One chest x-ray.
Drinking water that contains 5 parts per billion TCE (i.e., the TCE concentration equals its MCL) at a rate of 2 liters per day for 70 years.

Source of data used in table: Richard Wilson, "Analyzing the Daily Risks of Life," *Technology Review* (February 1979).

determine the MCLs for drinking water. So, as noted in Table 7, these commonplace activities produce risks equal to a *lifetime* consumption of drinking water at 5 µg/L TCE. Public pressures have demanded that the drinking water risk be no larger; but to date there has been no clamoring for restrictions on car travel or wine drinking (although the latter was tried, for very different reasons, during Prohibition). It is clear from Table 7 that the public accepts some risks much more readily than others.

So, is the public simply being difficult? What are the reasons for these differing risk perceptions? There have been many studies designed to assess this question, and the results are quite consistent. Table 8 lists some of the factors that seem to come into play in the overestimation or underestimation of risk.[57] Several of these factors when grouped together (fatal, personally at risk, not controllable, and not observable) give rise to a level of public fear that might be termed *dread*. It appears that the widespread public fear of cancer has reached this level, and it probably accounts for the strong public pressure for strict environmental standards. In demanding these standards, the public may be trying to exert control on the only part of the cancer problem that it sees as controllable.

The question is whether the level of control the public demands is

Table 8   Factors controlling risk perception and risk aversion.

Risk Perception	
Risks Overestimated	Risks Underestimated
Catastrophic	Not catastrophic
Fatal	Not fatal
Personally at risk	Not personally at risk
Risk not controllable	Risk controllable
Involuntary	Voluntary
Immediate	Delayed
Human-made	Natural
New risk	Old risk
Risk increasing	Risk decreasing
Not easily reduced	Easily reduced
Unfamiliar	Familiar
Unknown to science	Known to science
Not observable	Observable
Risk averse	Not risk averse

Risk Aversion

reasonable. About one out of four of us will die of cancer. In other words, the *background risk* that any one of us will sooner or later contract cancer is about 25 percent. By demanding that the *incremental risk* due to carcinogenic chemicals be kept to 1 in 1 million, or 0.0001 percent, the public is trying to prevent the total risk from increasing from 25 percent to 25.0001 percent. In a population of a million, this would imply 250,001 cases of cancer rather than 250,000. It is very questionable whether such small incremental risks are meaningful or measurable.[58]

The other factor in Table 8 that greatly influences dread is the perceived potential for catastrophic loss of life.[59] Experts and laypeople usually differ both with respect to the probability of such events and their likely consequences. This undoubtedly accounts for the generally strong level of support for nuclear power in the technical community and the strong opposition to it from a large segment of the public. Mind you, the public is more likely to accept nuclear risks if they are linked to jobs and economic growth. When Ralph Nader visited Richland, Washington, a city that depends on the nearby Hanford Nuclear Reservation for its economic health, he was greeted by 500 demonstrators waving placards reading "I Live in Richland and I Don't Glow in the Dark."[60] (Another pronuclear—and politically incorrect—bumper sticker observed in Richland: "Three Mile Island Is Better Built Than Jane Fonda.") It is likely that workers in the chemical industry have similar biases although I don't know of any studies that prove it.

The concept of risk aversion is closely associated with that of risk perception. On the basis of data like those shown in Tables 6 and 7, experts see the public as unreasonably averse to many risks, including those associated with nuclear power and environmental contamination. The most contentious risks are those for which the relative perceptions differ most. As suggested in Table 8, the same factors that control perception of risk also control aversion to risk.

Risk aversion can be put in an economic context. It is the extra amount of money that a decision maker is willing to spend in an effort to reduce a risk over and above the amount that represents the best estimate of the actual expenditure required. For the case of a landfill, it is the extra margin of safety that the owner-operator is willing to buy to avoid a future landfill failure (or at least one that will occur during the owner-operator's economic time horizon). For the public, in our context, it is the extra margin of protection that it demands to reduce health risks from environmental chemicals. Landfill owners tend to be somewhat risk-averse in their engineering designs. The public tends to be very risk-averse in its demands for environmental protection (or at least that follows from the deliberations of this chapter).

The question of what constitutes an *acceptable risk* is not a technical question; it is a social one. For each individual, it depends on risk perception, risk aversion, economic status, values, and beliefs. For the body politic, it is some type of integrated sum of these individual acceptable risks. It is not a fixed or known quantity. It is determined by the democratic process through elections, referendums, and public hearings, and under the influence of adversarial lobbies. It is the level at which "the political pressure dies down or the budget runs out."[61] It is determined by common consent, not by any sophisticated analysis. It sounds like a tautology, but acceptable risk is the risk associated with the most acceptable decision.[62]

In the environmental climate of recent years the carcinogenic risk of 1 in 1 million represents the acceptable risk because there has been no serious attempt to repeal it. It is worth noting, however, that in the site-specific risk-analysis procedures described earlier in this chapter, the EPA's regulations (and those of many state agencies as well) actually allow acceptable risks in the range 10^{-6} to 10^{-4} (i.e., from 1 in 1 million to 1 in 10,000). To date, regulatory personnel have been loathe to accept any calculated risk higher than 1 in 1 million, but in the last couple of years there have been hints of a movement toward larger acceptable risks.[63]

Kristin Shrader-Frechette, in her book *Risk and Rationality*, warns against all this talk of experts and laypeople.[64] She points out that experts may be just as susceptible to overconfidence about their risk predictions as are laypeople susceptible to their supposed irrational fears. She argues that all risks are "perceived," expert as well as lay. In her view, it is not possible to separate "perceived risk" from "actual risk," because the actual risks are unknown. If they were known, she argues, they would be certain, and hence no longer risks.

In my opinion, this populist perspective is not without merit. However, I do not accept the implication that there are no experts. All of us know more about some things than our fellows, whether it be how to prune roses, play a bridge hand, or tie a fishing fly. This is no less so for issues of risk. Now, it may be true that in a democratic society government tends to respond as much to public perceptions as to the proclamations of experts. But I do not think that recognizing the importance of public perceptions absolves the experts from the responsibility to inform the public of *their* perceptions of the risks facing humankind. Public policy has large price tags associated with it, and the public ought to be fully informed on the extra costs it is bearing to achieve the risk reductions it desires.

PLAYING GOD: THE DOLLAR VALUE OF LIFE

There is something seamy about trying to place a dollar value on life, health, and happiness. As E. F. Schumacher put it in his wise and influential book *Small Is Beautiful*, "To undertake to measure the unmeasurable is absurd. The higher is reduced to the level of the lower and the priceless is given a price."[65]

Well, maybe so, but ethical quagmire though it may be, it seems difficult to avoid trying to convert health risks into dollar values so that we have a rational context for assessing alternative policies for managing environmental contamination. Despite the murky waters, it is hard to avoid placing a dollar value on life.

Take dam construction, for example. Every time a dam is built, the downstream residents are put at risk. If the dam should fail, there will be catastrophic loss of life and property. The dam designers, of course, take this eventuality into account in their design, but as I discussed earlier, even the best engineering designs have some small probability of failure attached to them. This probability of failure can be decreased by building ever more safety into the design, but increased safety involves increased costs, and at some point the dam designer (or the dam owner) will decide that enough is enough. There is no way around it: in this process they are trading dollars for risk. They could spend more and decrease the risk, or spend less and increase the risk. And because the risk includes possible loss of life, they are trading dollars for lives (at least in a probabilistic sense).

This same reasoning process can be applied to public policy. Environmental regulations that protect public health and safety also have a cost associated with them. There are direct costs to the taxpayer for the implementation and enforcement of the regulations, and there are costs to the regulated community that are usually passed on to the consumer in the form of higher product prices. As with dams, there are increasing costs associated with increasing risk reduction. The more you spend, the more lives you will save. So once again we are forced to think the unthinkable and place value on life.

There is a huge amount of literature on the value of life, both philosophical and practical. Much of it comes from the insurance industry, where putting value on life is a business. Regardless of the context, all studies of life valuation are quick to point out that we are not valuing a specific life, yours or mine, but rather a statistical life, a faceless life that does not belong to anyone you know. It is a dodge to be sure, but it seems a necessary one.

In the life valuation literature there are five approaches that have been used to estimate the value of a statistical life.[66] The first is the human productivity approach, which is based on the net present worth of future lost earnings of someone whose life is lost. The second is a legal approach based on court awards in negligence cases involving loss of life. The third is an implicit evaluation based on the willingness to pay for reduced risk as evidenced by the existence of risk-compensating wage differentials and pollution-related differentials in property values. The fourth is based on the consumption by the public of life-saving goods and services like smoke alarms and air bags. The last is a de facto valuation based on the value of life implicitly embedded in government regulations already enacted.

Table 9 indicates the results of a review carried out by one set of researchers for four of these five approaches.[67] There are two conclusions that emerge from perusal of this table. First, estimates of the value of life cover a very wide range, from as little as $57,000 to more than $10 million. And second, the $10 million figure looks like a kind of upper bound. You undoubtedly feel that your own life is infinitely valuable, but a statistical life is apparently worth no more than $10 million, and on average much less.

There are of course lots of problems, ethical and otherwise, with each of these methods. Given current income statistics, the human productivity approach would value the life of a white-collar worker higher than that of a blue-collar worker, and a man more than a woman. The legal approach places us at the whim of a jury. The three implicit valuations seem a little less loaded, and perhaps the de facto valuation embedded in government regulations is as good an approach as any. The public acceptance of a government regulation that involves health or safety is a measure of the politically acceptable limit to the number of statistical lives that the public is willing to leave at risk.

If the value of life is to be a component of the risk term in a risk–cost-

Table 9   Summary of some calculations of the value of life.

Approach	Number of Studies	Range of Values ($US)
Human productivity approach	4	$378,000–$2.82 million
Court awards in legal cases[a]	—	——
Willingness of people to pay for reduced risk	8	$57,000–$10.1 million
Consumption of life-saving goods and services	4	$180,000–$466,000
De facto valuation in government regulations	3	$227,000–$9.45 million

[a]Data not available.

Source of data used in table: Mark Sharefkin, Mordechai Schecter, and Allen Kneese, "Impacts, Costs, and Techniques for Mitigation of Contaminated Groundwater: A Review," *Water Resources Research* 20 (1984): 1771–83.

benefit assessment, then a point made earlier is worth repeating. It is inappropriate to discount dollars and lives at the same discount rate.[68] The value of money varies over time; the value of life does not. It is advisable to keep dollars and lives in separate accounts (even if the value of life has been converted to dollars) so that they can be discounted (or not discounted) at the appropriate rates.

Life-saving regulations often involve trade-offs. I have noted, for example, that the practice of introducing chlorine into drinking-water supplies produces organic chemicals in the water that create a small, incremental risk of cancer. The risk involved, however, is orders of magnitude lower than the risk removed by the chlorination, that associated with pathogenic microorganisms. Immunization provides another example. Out of the 3.5 million children annually immunized against whooping cough, diphtheria, and tetanus, about 20 die each year.[69] It is a tragic way to lose a child, yet public health services (and apparently the public, too) find these risks preferable to the frequent incidence of disease and death that would occur without immunization programs.

These examples involve looking at the pluses and minuses within specific life-saving programs. The alternative courses of action are relatively simple. Either we chlorinate the water (or immunize the children) or we don't. If the step will lead to a net reduction in risk, it is worthy of consideration. More difficult trade-offs arise when we try to compare risk reduction across a suite of different life-saving programs, or across a suite of different health-enhancing regulations, that involve different risks. This is the world of priority setting, and it raises the thorny question of *whose* risk we should choose to reduce.

SETTING PRIORITIES: NEEDLES, CONDOMS, AND CLEAN WATER

There is an upper bound on the tax revenues that governments can expect to extract from their citizens. Liberals and conservatives can argue about what that limit is, but clearly it is finite. In this situation (which is the only situation there is), there is an unavoidable competition for social resources. How much government revenue should be spent on health and safety, relative to that spent on, say, inner-city poverty or improvement of the racial milieu? Of that portion earmarked for health and safety, how much should go to sanitation, AIDS, or the Superfund? Within an environmental framework, how should we apportion resources between the protection of water quality and the protection of air quality? Governments have an unavoidable need to prioritize, and the public has an unavoidable obligation to provide direction.

When it comes to health and safety regulations, society would be able to provide better direction if it had a better handle on what level of risk reduction can be achieved with the various proposed or existing regulations, so that it can decide whether the achievable risk reductions are worth the cost. It is always hard to predict the impact of proposed regulations, but it is quite feasible to look at the performance of existing regulations. Data exist on annual costs; and, while difficult, it is possible to estimate the annual number of lives saved by a given regulation. With this information in hand, it is possible to determine the resulting cost per life saved. Table 10 is based on a study that compared forty-four U.S. health and safety regulations through 1986 as to cost per life saved.[70]

Table 10 Cost per life saved for a selection of risk-reducing regulations.

Regulation	Year	Agency	Annual Lives Saved	Cost per Life Saved ($US)
Steering column protection	1967	NHTSA	1300	100
Seat cushion flammability	1984	FAA	37	600
Children's sleepwear flammability	1973	CPSC	106	1,300
Benzene emissions	1984	EPA	0.31	2,800
Arsenic levels in glass plants	1986	EPA	0.11	19,200
Radionuclides at DOE facilities	1984	EPA	0.001	210,000
Land disposal	1986	EPA	2.5	3,500,000
Pesticide EDB	1983	OSHA	0.002	15,600,000

Source of data used in table: John F. Morrall III, "A Review of the Record," *Regulation* (November-December 1986), as quoted in Howard Holme, "Risk Assessment and Cost-Benefit Analysis Are Keys to Environmental Law Reform" (American Society of Civil Engineers 22nd Annual Conference, Cambridge, Mass., May 9, 1995).

The range of values is astounding, from $100 per life saved, for an auto safety regulation, to more than $15 million per life saved, for regulation of the pesticide ethylene dibromide. The land disposal regulation of 1986 listed in Table 10, which cost $3.5 million per life saved, is not identified in detail, but it is likely related to RCRA or Superfund rule making.

In general, auto safety regulations are more effective than environmental regulations in saving lives. Referring to the same study, another author notes that with a $1 billion budget for risk reduction, one could save 2,000 lives through auto safety regulations or 27 lives through cancer-oriented environmental protection.[71]

Many authors make the argument that life extension is a better metric than lives saved.[72] Most people ascribe a large value to healthy increased longevity, perhaps even more than they would give to protect against sudden unexpected loss of life. In this case the effectiveness measure for regulations becomes the cost per year of increased longevity, rather than the cost per life saved. A study by the Harvard Center for Risk Analysis looked at 587 life-enhancing interventions from this perspective.[73] They grouped the various types of interventions into categories and then calculated the median cost per year of increased longevity for each category. For interventions that lead to fatal-injury reduction, they found the median cost to be on the order of $50,000 per year of increased longevity. For interventions involving toxin control, they calculated a cost of more than $2 million. Once again, health-protecting environmental regulations aimed at control of toxic chemicals fared very poorly relative to regulations that provide more direct impact on health and safety.

Richard Schwing, coeditor of the book *Societal Risk Assessment: How Safe Is Safe Enough?* suggests that a diagram like Figure 9 can be informative.[74] This figure indicates the effectiveness of various health and safety measures by plotting the estimated increase in longevity provided by the measure against the cost per year of increased longevity. He does not include the cleanup of contaminated sites in the suite of measures he assesses (of which only a few are shown in Figure 9), but it is clear that such cleanups would be plotted near the upper boundary of the diagram where cost effectiveness is low.

In an in-house EPA study of Superfund costs in the New England states, the cost per statistical life saved at "high-risk sites" fell into the range $340,000–$7.7 million,[75] which would appear to be in the range indicated in Table 9 for the value of life. "Low-risk sites," on the other hand, came in at $3–7 billion per life saved, which is orders of magnitude higher than the highest value on that table. On the basis of this assessment, it would seem that only the highest-risk Superfund sites are cost effective in the sense of saving lives, and even these are at the high end in terms of cost per life saved.

Sometimes in preparing this material, I felt like I was drowning in a sea of statistics. One day I decided to look into the trenches of real life, so I called up a public health officer who works the mean streets in my home city. When I asked him about the impact of contaminated sites he just scoffed. "My life is drug addicts and AIDS victims," he said. "We're going to lose a bunch of kids on the streets next year and nobody seems to care. In most cases, it's for lack of clean needles and condoms." He thought for a minute. "You know, your suburbanites are willing to

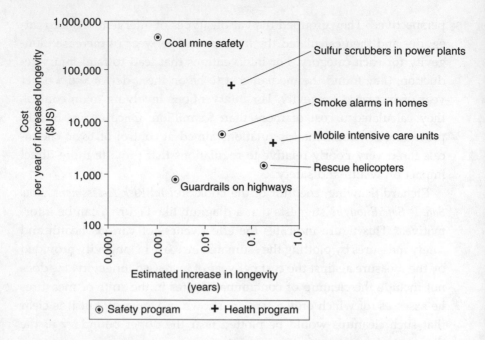

Figure 9. Effectiveness of a variety of health and safety measures. (Source of data used in figure: Richard C. Schwing, "Trade-Offs," in *Societal Risk Assessment: How Safe Is Safe Enough?* ed. Richard C. Schwing and Walter A. Albers Jr. [New York: Plenum Press, 1980], 129–41.)

spend millions to protect themselves against a one-in-a-million shot of getting cancer. I could buy enough needles and condoms to last forever for a tenth the cost of one of your cleanups."

THE SOCIAL COSTS OF OVERKILL AND UNDERKILL

John A. Hird, in his book *Superfund: The Political Economy of Environmental Risk,* estimates that more than 90 percent of mainstream scientists do not regard chemical hazardous waste as a major long-term environmental health threat. He sees this difference with public opinion as a fundamental public policy problem.[76] Robert Raucher, a noted water resource economist, asks: Given the asymmetries in perceived risk, "whose views should determine policy—the experts' or the public's? . . . If the public is really misinformed we have a dilemma as to whether we ignore the public and follow the experts, or blindly follow the public even though we know they're misinformed."[77]

In 1987, the EPA carried out an in-house evaluation of the relative risks of a wide range of environmental problems and published the results in a report entitled *Unfinished Business*.[78] The agency found that the EPA's priorities more closely mirrored the public's perception of risks than that of the experts. If one believes that the risk perceptions of the experts are more reliable than those of the public, then one would conclude that the EPA programs are putting too much emphasis on Superfund sites and not enough on the questions of ozone depletion and global warming. The in-house study concluded that too much of the EPA's resource base was going to issues of local site contamination and not enough to larger global questions.

Three years later, there was a follow-up study by the EPA's quasi-independent Science Advisory Board. In their report *Reducing Risk*, the board's members divided environmental risks into those associated with ecology and welfare and those associated with human health.[79] Under the latter heading they limited themselves to more local pollution problems. They rated as "high risks": air pollution, occupational chemical exposure, indoor pollutants including radon, and lead contamination of drinking water as a result of the use of plumbing systems with lead pipes and solder. They listed groundwater pollution, which has turned out to be the primary target of the Superfund and RCRA programs as a "low risk."

If these assessments are correct, then it is clear that the over-expenditure of resources in these latter programs is creating a shortage of resources in areas of greater need. In this period of retrenchment, where the total funds directed to environmental issues are likely to shrink rather than grow, the unavoidable consequence of overkill in one area is underkill in another.

The trade-off between expenditures on air pollution and water pollution, particularly as the latter relates to hazardous-waste sites, is a particularly touchy one. Currently, much more is spent on water than air, primarily due to the high cost of the Superfund. Yet in November 1996, when the EPA published its proposed new national air quality regulations, it claimed that the new standards would prevent 15,000 premature deaths each year.[80] No water-quality regulations related to contaminated-site cleanup could come close to these numbers. Expert panels, within the EPA and outside of it, have consistently rated air pollution as a greater health hazard than water pollution.[81]

However, public opinion has just as consistently put it the other way around. It is not clear why the public is so sanguine with respect to air pollution. Perhaps, like smoking and car accidents, it is simply too familiar. Maybe the issue has become too closely connected to Los Angeles in people's minds, and the rest of the country figures those Hollywood moguls deserve what they get. Certainly, anyone who drives into the dark haze of Los Angeles (or many other large American cities) on a perfectly sunny day must wonder what kind of fumes and particulates they are drawing into their lungs with every breath.

If there is overkill in the regulation and remediation of contaminated sites, how might we correct the situation? There are several possibilities: (1) The MCLs could be raised for some chemicals, thus removing many marginally contaminated sites that pose negligible health risk from consideration for remedial action. (2) It could be recognized that drinking-water MCLs are inappropriate as triggers for remedial action at contaminated sites and alternative criteria could be put in place. (3) Protocols for quantitative risk assessments could be reviewed, with an eye to removing some of the many overconservative assumptions. (4) The 1 in 1 million level of acceptable risk could be softened. (5) Priority-setting protocols based on cost per life saved or cost per year of increased longevity could be put in place to compare proposed alternative life-saving and health-enhancing regulations.

It is worth noting that these suggestions do not include a call for the repeal of contaminated-sites regulations. As discussed in chapter 2, given the economic pressures placed on the corporate decision makers, it is unlikely that without the presence of environmental legislation and enforcement they would find it possible to implement policies that guarantee environmental protection. What is needed now is not repeal of the strides we have made toward environmental respectability, but rather a fine-tuning of the application of the laws to avoid remedial overkill. The gray hats of corporate America still need protection from themselves.

I started this chapter by trying to determine what really matters with respect to environmental contamination. I hope it is now becoming clear that what really matters is not just a question of which chemicals are present at a site and how toxic they are, but that it's also a question of the site-specific potential for human exposure and health degradation. Attempts to enforce universal laws with standardized protocols are bound to fail. There is no alternative to site-specific regulatory enforcement.

There are three main pathways by which contamination of sites may lead to local health degradation: (1) direct contact with contaminants, (2) use of groundwater from contaminated aquifers, and (3) use of surface water from rivers or other contaminated surface-water bodies. Back in Figure 6 I identified the locations of a number of the worst contamination incidents in North America. In Table 11 the nature of the exposure pathway at twenty of these sites is summarized. Two of the sites (Love Canal and Times Beach) involved direct contact; six of the sites contaminated drinking-water aquifers; and ten of the sites discharged contaminated water into rivers or other surface-water bodies. However, of these last ten, only two produced contaminated concentrations in the rivers that were large enough to measure. In the other eight cases, the rate of delivery of contaminated mass to the rivers was so small that its dilution by the river flow made it impossible to even detect, let alone lead to the risk of health degradation. There is a long-standing credo in the environmental world that "dilution is no solution to pollution," and certainly it should never be used *by design* as a part of the solution. However, in cases of historical contamination, it seems somehow foolish to demand the expenditure of social resources for site remediation if nature is providing the solution for free.

If one accepts this argument, then approximately half of the twenty sites in Table 11 require the application of stringent drinking-water standards as a remedial trigger, and the other half would be candidates for less-stringent criteria. Table 11 covers twenty of the *worst* contaminated

Table 11 Impacts of contaminated sites.

Number of Major Contaminated Sites in Figure 6	20
Number of sites where health impacts due to direct contact with contaminants have been documented.	2
Number of sites that have contaminated a drinking-water aquifer, or threaten to do so.	6
Number of sites that discharge contaminants to rivers or other surface-water bodies, or threaten to do so.	10
Of those sites that discharge contaminants to surface water, number of sites that lead to measurable surface-water contaminant concentrations.	2

sites in North America. If one were to include the thousands of contaminated sites currently under regulatory control, including the marginal ones as well as the worst ones, I have little doubt that the number of sites that would prove eligible for the less-stringent action levels would climb from 50 percent to 90 percent or more.

The environmental movement deserves the credit for alerting us all to a wide range of environmental risks. It is largely responsible for the current level of dedication to environmental protection in North America. However, as a movement, it is experiencing the same problems that other movements have experienced when the time comes for new paradigms. It continues to fight the local battles where support is easy to come by, even though the marginal risks associated with newly emerging sites get smaller and smaller. The movement could play a more valuable role if it would try to inform the public about the relative risks associated with different issues and try to lead the public to take a greater interest in some of the higher-risk issues. Many of these issues, such as ozone depletion and global warming, require a more global vision, and it has historically been more difficult to garner meaningful support from the public to address the types of risk that do not pose an immediate local threat.

Even in the case of contaminated sites, the greatest risks now lie outside our country, as evidenced by the shocking environmental revelations from behind the old Iron Curtain after the fall of Communism in eastern Europe. Chernobyl is simply the tip of an eastern European iceberg of environmental degradation. As noted by Jay Lehr, "Rather than chasing smaller and smaller amounts of less and less important substances in our own country, environmentalists should now address their attention to those parts of the world in greater need, to help them achieve the success we in America already enjoy."[82]

Thanks to the warnings of the environmental movement, the social costs of underkill are well recognized. They include environmental degradation and unacceptable impacts on human health. The social costs of overkill are less well recognized. They include diversion of resources from areas of greater need, unwarranted emphasis on remediation of past mistakes rather than prevention of future ones, reduction of trust in government action, and misuse of science and technology. The enforcement of regulations that lead to environmental overkill also create a host of ethical conundrums for all concerned, whether they be corporate decision makers, technical consultants, or government regulators. In the remaining chapters I will examine some of the causes of overkill and underkill and explore the nature of some of the social costs.

THE BOTTOM LINE

- There is a suite of chemicals, composed primarily of chlorinated organics and metals, known to be toxic and/or carcinogenic when experienced in acute doses by human beings exposed during industrial accidents or by small animals exposed during laboratory experimentation.

- There is considerable controversy in the scientific community about how to extrapolate the evidence from acute exposures to applications involving chronic environmental exposures, and from animal data to human dose-response relationships. With the current level of available data, there appears to be an irreducible degree of uncertainty as to the level of risk associated with long-term, low-dose, chronic environmental exposures to toxic chemicals.

- The maximum contaminant levels put in place by the EPA to ensure protection against human carcinogenic or noncarcinogenic impacts resulting from chronic environmental chemical exposure are extremely conservative. Despite current uncertainties, it is likely that most organic MCLs could be raised by an order of magnitude (or perhaps more) without harm to human health.

- Even if it were decided that the current MCLs are appropriate for regulating the potability of public water supplies, it is now clear that they are inappropriate as a trigger for remedial action at contaminated sites that do not threaten drinking-water sources.

- The alternative approach using quantitative risk assessment of offsite risks as the trigger for action at contaminated sites is superior in principle to the perfunctory application of MCLs at on-site monitoring wells. However, the assumptions inherent in the current protocols and the use of unrealistic receptor scenarios has led to a situation where the health risks from contaminated sites are significantly overestimated, perhaps by as much as two orders of magnitude.

- The public perceives risks associated with environmental chemicals and contaminated sites to be higher than "experts" in environmental risk perceive them to be. Objective assessments of the cost per life saved, or the cost per year of increased longevity, of a wide suite of risk-reducing regulations indicate that environmental regulations aimed at control of toxic chemicals are less effective than regulations that provide more direct impact on health and safety.

- *What really matters* at contaminated sites is not just a question of which chemicals are present and how toxic they are, but also of the sometimes-limited potential for human exposure. Current environmental policies overemphasize remedial action at contaminated sites. There are social costs associated with such overkill, not the least of which is the diversion of resources from other environmental programs that address issues of greater risk, including air pollution, ozone depletion, and global warming.

- There remains a need for contaminated-sites regulation. Simplistic calls for the repeal of environmental legislation in a Contract-with-America sense are extremely dangerous. What is needed is not abandonment of the legislation, but fine-tuning of the *application* of the legislation to avoid remedial overkill.

4 The Unpleasant Truths about Waste Management

Even if we accept the conclusions of the previous chapter, that the level of human health risk engendered by historical contamination has been somewhat overblown, we are still left with the uncomfortable facts of environmental carelessness. When it comes to environmental steward-ship of the land, our legacy of past sins appears unforgivable. The work ethic and human ingenuity that have made the United States and Canada among the richest nations on earth have been brought to bear in great measure on the developmental end of the product cycles, where the prof-its are made, but they have not extended to the back end where the waste streams emerge and there are only costs to be borne. We have been lazy, and we have sullied our landscape with contamination.

Some of the alarming statistics have already been thrown at you. We have generated hundreds of millions of tons of hazardous industrial waste per year for many years past, much of it charged with toxic and carcinogenic metals and organic chemicals. The great majority of it has ended up in tens of thousands of industrial landfills and waste lagoons, most of which are unlined, unmonitored, and incapable of stopping waste leachates from migrating offsite into groundwater, wetlands, and streams.

It is reasonable to ask how this state of affairs came to pass. How could a country with the technical capabilities to send a man to the moon be incapable of recognizing these threats to the nation's environmental health?

THE PAST:
MALICIOUS INTENT OR JUST PLAIN DUMB?

There are some who would argue that the waste disposal strategies of the forties, fifties, and sixties were premeditated and malicious, carried out by corporate America in full knowledge of their environmental consequences and for the sole purpose of enhancing bottom-line profits. This historical interpretation leads logically to the argument that current regulatory policies should be punitive with respect to the parties responsible for past contamination. Indeed, as we shall see, there *is* a strong punitive element in the Superfund legislation, so it can be assumed that the framers of this legislation accepted this viewpoint, at least to some degree.

I do not subscribe to this capitalist-conspiracy theory of environmental contamination. In the first place, environmental contamination in the postwar years is a phenomenon common to all the developed countries of the world regardless of their political persuasion or economic system. It is now clear that environmental degradation behind the Iron Curtain is far worse than on this side of it, despite the presumably greater degree of government control on industry there and the stronger presence of centralized planning inherent in a socialist system. In the second place, naive though it may appear, I just can't conjure up the necessary level of amorality in the boardrooms of America to support the evil cabal scenario. I believe that the real explanation is more prosaic. The issue is ignorance and indifference, not malicious intent.

Waste disposal in the forties and fifties still reflected an out-of-sight, out-of-mind mentality. Many coastal cities still dumped much of their waste into the ocean from barges offshore. Hazardous liquid wastes were often injected into deep wells to an uncertain subsurface fate. Dumps were sited in abandoned pits (witness Ville Mercier and the Love Canal), or worse yet, in swamps, which were then still regarded as wastelands of little value to society. The civil engineers who designed waste-management facilities had little or no training in geology and hydrology. The ultimate fate of leachates that might drain out the bottom of unlined landfills simply did not come under consideration. The nature of groundwater flow systems was not understood in the engineering community, nor was there sufficient realization of the linkage between groundwater and surface water systems.

On the other side of the fence, geologists and hydrologists who *were* familiar with groundwater and surface water flow were almost totally engaged in the development of water resources for public water supply. They were not asked to participate in waste-management decisions and did not recognize the relevance of their expertise to such decisions. Even as late as 1980, in the major journals dedicated to groundwater science and engineering there was essentially no discussion of the contamination of groundwater by dissolved chlorinated solvents.[1]

In those early years, water samples were often analyzed for their potability, but the target contaminants were those associated with sewage and human waste, for which there was a long history of sanitation issues. The threat associated with the new organic chemicals had to await Rachel Carson's clarion call in 1962. Even then, it was not until many years later, in the late seventies and early eighties, that suitable analytical methods became available in the laboratory for the routine identification of industrial organic chemicals in water. Only then did the scale of the problem emerge. The contamination of drinking water with chlorinated solvents was reported from cities around the country. Among the earliest and most influential findings were those from Long Island, New York; Bedford, Massachusetts; New Orleans, Louisiana; and the San Gabriel and Santa Clara Valleys of California. A detailed historical study of this period identifies the end of 1981 as "the milestone for the end of the period of general ignorance of the fact that poor [chemical] handling practices and careless disposal can cause severe contamination of groundwater."[2]

Evidence of the ignorance of the early years, and the slowly emerging understanding of the problem, can be seen in Table 12, which reproduces the disposal instructions for solvents such as TCE and methylene chloride provided on Chemical Safety Data Sheets issued over the period 1968 to 1980 by the Manufacturing Chemists Association and other groups.[3] Their early recommendations for disposal created solvent releases into the environment that are identical to the ones we now spend millions of dollars trying to avoid.

In hindsight, the late awareness of the hazards posed to the environment by organic chemicals from industrial operations and waste disposal practices can be seen as a failure of several segments of modern society: government regulation, industrial practice, and environmental research.[4] In the early years, the cause of the failure was ignorance, and a lack of communication across the disciplines. It is unlikely that there was widespread malicious intent on the part of any of the players. Perhaps in the later years, one cannot let corporate America off the hook so easily. Even after 1981, by which time the dimensions of the problem were clear, corporations were very slow to respond. Studies of individual cases invariably indicate considerable concern over disposal practices at the working level long before management was cajoled into taking appropriate action.[5] Not only that, but as we shall see in later chapters, once the hammer of the Superfund was brought down in 1980, there is no question that many corporations stonewalled the EPA's initiatives because of bottom-line worries. It is possible that the harsh punitive features of the Superfund engendered this defensive response. Members of the new right will undoubtedly embrace this interpretation; environmentalists will scoff; and the rest of us are left to wonder how industry would have reacted to a softer, more cooperative approach.

Table 12 Disposal instructions for solvents on Chemical Safety Data Sheets issued by the Manufacturing Chemists Association and other industry groups over the period 1968–1980.

Year	Disposal Instruction
1968	[Solvents] "may be poured on dry sand, earth, or ashes . . . and allowed to evaporate into the atmosphere."
1971	"Bury [the solvents] away from water supply or allow solvent to evaporate to atmosphere at a safe distance from inhabited buildings."
1973	"In some cases, small amounts [of the solvent] can be transported to an area where it can be placed on the ground and allowed to evaporate."
1979	"In some cases, small amounts [of the solvent] can be transported to an area where it can be placed on the ground and allowed to evaporate safely if local, state, and federal regulations permit."
1980	"Dumping [of solvents] into sewers, on the ground, or into any body of water is strongly discouraged, and may be illegal."

Source of information used in table: J. F. Pankow, Stan Feenstra, John A. Cherry, and M. Cathryn Ryan, "Dense Chlorinated Solvents in Groundwater: Background and History of the Problem," in *Dense Chlorinated Solvents and Other DNAPLs in Groundwater: History, Behavior, and Remediation,* ed. J. F. Pankow and John A. Cherry (Waterloo, Ont.: Waterloo Press, 1996).

REMEDIATION OR PREVENTION? SHOULD WE EMPHASIZE THE CORRECTION OF PAST MISTAKES OR THE PREVENTION OF FUTURE ONES?

There is an unavoidable connection between waste management and environmental protection. The methods we use to manage our waste will in large part control the degree of environmental protection that we can achieve. Putting this statement in a more economic framework: the costs we are willing to bear for waste management will control the benefits that are likely to accrue from environmental protection. It is difficult to achieve political consensus on this trade-off because the costs are in terms of real dollars while the benefits are in terms of aesthetic pleasure and improved health. Left to their own devices individual companies are likely to try to minimize their waste disposal costs at the expense of the social benefits of environmental protection. In response, the public at large has demanded legislation that drives the companies toward a more socially acceptable position. In the United States these demands led to the formation of the Environmental Protection Agency and ultimately to development of two different types of legislation for environmental protection. The first, represented by the Superfund legislation, is designed to force responsible parties to clean up their past mistakes. It is the remediation option. The second, represented by the RCRA legislation, is designed to prevent future contamination from industrial sites. It is the prevention option. One of the thorniest issues legislators and regulatory agencies face in trying to establish effective environmental policy is deciding on the optimal mix of prevention and remediation.

The importance of remediation in the mix depends in part on one's perception of the magnitude of the problem. The EPA's internal estimate of the total number of potential Superfund sites has varied over the years, but most recent estimates have hovered around 30,000 sites. Of these, the number with "obvious hazardous release problems," and thus worthy of being placed on the National Priorities List (NPL), has grown from initial estimates of fewer than 1,000 to recent estimates of the likelihood of 2,000 sites by the turn of the century. Of course the Chemical Manufacturers Association, representing industrial interests, sees things somewhat differently, recognizing only 4,800 potential sites and only 400 NPL candidates. On the other side of the environmental spectrum, the National Audubon Society worries that there might be as many as 7,000 NPL sites.[6]

Whatever number one chooses to use, it is clear that the number of sites that are actually going to see meaningful remedial effort is quite small relative to the total number of contaminated sites thought to exist around the nation. The fact is that there are just too many sites, and it is simply not economically feasible to attack them all. Worse yet, as we shall see in chapter 5, there are technical problems at the sites undergoing cleanup. Cleanup is not proceeding smoothly, and there are those who now think that much of the attempted remediation is technically as well as economically infeasible.

This situation has led many to espouse a greater role for prevention of contamination in environmental policy. John Cherry of the University of Waterloo, one of North America's leading experts on contaminated sites, decries the current focus on the restoration of a relatively small number of industrial sites and argues that the focus of environmental policy should be on prevention of contamination rather than remediation. He notes that the cost of removal of one pound of contaminant mass from subsurface soils and groundwater is "immense" in comparison to adapting industrial facilities and procedures to prevent the entry of contaminants into the subsurface.[7] Charles Job of the EPA states that "dealing with contamination may be 30 to 40 times more costly than preventing it in the first place."[8]

In the United States the primary legislative effort aimed at the prevention of environmental pollution is the Resource Conservation and Recovery Act, first passed in 1976 and subsequently amended in 1984. Like most laws dealing with technically complex topics, it specifies goals in general terms and then directs the appropriate agency, in this case the EPA, to stipulate the exact requirements in the form of legally binding regulations and nonbinding guidance documents.

RCRA mandates a cradle-to-grave program for the management of hazardous industrial waste. It requires the operators of waste-disposal facilities to use state-of-the-art design features, carry out careful monitoring programs to ensure that the facility is functioning as designed, and have corrective-action contingency plans in place should anything go wrong.[9]

RCRA has had a somewhat rocky history, and little was accomplished in the first eight years or so after its passage. The Hazardous and Solid Waste Amendments (HSWA) to RCRA in 1984 were actually a congressional slap on the wrist for the perceived lack of action on the part of the EPA and the foot-dragging of the Reagan administration on environmental matters. The goal of the HSWA amendments was to discourage hazardous-waste landfills and encourage waste reduction at the source, in the industrial production processes. However, this has really never come to pass. While there have been some successes in industrial waste reduction, the successes have not been of sufficient magnitude to remove the need for land-based hazardous-waste disposal. Nor, if we are realistic about it, will they ever be. It is an unfortunate fact, but hazardous-waste landfills are here to stay, and even pie-in-the-sky congressional posturing will not make them go away.

If that is the case, then one might well ask the question: Could a RCRA landfill ever become a Superfund site? Or worded another way: Are the RCRA requirements sufficiently robust to prevent environmental releases that could lead to human health risk? It would be reassuring to get a positive answer to this latter question. Unfortunately, that is not the answer that comes out of a study carried out by the Office of Technology Assessment (OTA), the watchdog agency on technical matters for the U.S. Congress. The agency looked into this exact issue and came to a negative conclusion,[10] stating that "RCRA groundwater protection standards are not likely to prevent land disposal sites from becoming uncontrolled sites that will require cleanup under Superfund." In fact, as of 1984, 50 RCRA sites were already on the National Priorities List for the Superfund program; and in 1988, the EPA estimated that 800 leaking RCRA facilities might need to be transferred in due course to the Superfund program.

The OTA study identified some of the flaws in the RCRA legislation that have led to this pass. Primary among them was the fact that RCRA provisions stop at the fence line. There is no requirement to address offsite leakage outside the property line. Perhaps more important, monitoring requirements cease 30 years after site closure. This is much too soon. Operator liability ends at the very time when liner mortality curves suggest that landfill liners and caps are most likely to wear out.

Linda Greer of the Natural Resources Defense Council makes the further point that RCRA does not regulate a number of important waste streams.[11] For example, the mining industry and oil and gas production are explicitly exempted from RCRA. In addition, compliance is limited to a set of listed chemicals that does not include some of the worst actors from the pesticide production process.

Lastly, the issue of enforcement remains largely unresolved. Passing environmental laws is easy, but enforcing them is difficult and costly. It is one thing to keep your arms around a thousand sites, as the Superfund office has to do; it is another thing to enforce a law that aspires to regulate every industrial site in the country, tens of thousands of them, as RCRA purports to do. When thinking on the optimal remediation-prevention mix, the Achilles heel on the remediation side is technical feasibility, while on the prevention side it is administrative feasibility. Both have economic implications.

While critics may decry the flaws in the RCRA regulations, the fact is that we have come a long way. It is far from perfect, but the RCRA legislation has put American industry on notice that waste management must be carried out in a responsible fashion. Corporate America is slowly learning that the best way to avoid the wrath of the Superfund law is to prevent contaminant releases to the environment. This has led to many environmentally driven overhauls of old industrial plants, the institution of spill-prevention measures, redesign of pipeline and sewer systems, and a shift from belowground to aboveground tank storage. One can argue that full success has not yet been achieved, but the preventive philosophy of RCRA is taking hold, and with continued interaction between government and industry, some of it cooperative and some of it probably adversarial, continued improvement is almost certain.

In addition to RCRA, the EPA has a couple of other prevention instruments in its arsenal. Two programs mandated under the Safe Drinking Water Act serve to support the prevention of aquifer contamination.[12] In the Wellhead Protection Program, support is provided to local communities to delineate protection areas around public water-supply wells, and to develop and implement management plans that protect these areas from contamination. The Sole Source Aquifer Program prevents federal financial assistance to any project that may contaminate any aquifer designated as a principal drinking-water source. As of 1995, 65 regional aquifers had been so designated, including the New Jersey Coastal Plain aquifer, which serves 543,000 people, the Great Miami River Buried Valley aquifer in Ohio, which serves 921,000 people, and the Eastern Snake River Plain aquifer in Idaho, which serves 275,000 people. Between 1990 and 1995, 1,192 projects were reviewed by the EPA to assess their potential for contamination of sole-source aquifers. While only a few projects were not approved, many were modified to improve spill-containment measures, eliminate wastewater injection to the subsurface, and add monitoring networks.

These two programs do not represent a comprehensive policy for

protecting aquifer recharge areas, but they do provide a cost-effective
approach to the protection of public health. If we accept the premise that
prevention is a more viable approach to environmental protection than
remediation, then programs like these ought to be beefed up. Much of
the money currently being spent under the Superfund for remediation
of individual contaminated sites would be better spent on these regional
aquifer protection programs.

IS RECYCLING THE ANSWER?

In earlier chapters we have learned about the product cycles that un-
derlie the supply of material goods that make our lives livable, and the
ubiquitous generation of waste at every turn in these product cycles. We
have become aware of the huge waste loads that the environment is
forced to accept and looked at the statistics on the huge number of contaminated sites that result.

Surely, one asks, there must be a way to reduce these waste streams
and mitigate our insult to the land. What is the potential for waste reduction? Realistically, what can be achieved through recovery, reuse,
and recycling? In short: Is recycling the answer?

First of all, it is worth differentiating between the two main types of
recycling activities: those designed to reduce the load of nonhazardous
municipal waste that comes largely from household garbage, and those
designed to reduce the load of hazardous industrial waste streams. We
will look at each in turn.

Recycling of household garbage has been a central focus of the environmental movement since its birth, and there is no question that the
establishment of recycling centers and blue-box programs has raised the
awareness of the public regarding the value and importance of waste
reduction and recovery. In one sense, these programs have simply
tapped into the fundamental human inclination toward thrift and fru-
gality. There has always been informal commercial trade in used goods,
like furniture, appliances, and cars. Who among us can ignore the allure
of a good old-fashioned junk store? Every weekend, the antique malls,

flea markets, garage sales, and thrift shops of the nation are flooded with bargain hunters and curiosity seekers. Every automobile junkyard serves a vast underground community of dealers and traders in used car parts. The embracement of recycling by the public is in the same spirit of bartering and sharing that has always been an essential part of Americana.

Household recycling programs have largely been aimed at keeping the least biodegradable items out of municipal landfills: glass bottles, plastic containers, metal cans, and newspaper. Volunteer organizations and service groups have raised cash for years through collection and recycling of these commodities. I still remember fondly the Boy Scout newspaper drives of my youth. In recent years, much of this effort has become more formalized through blue-box curbside pickup programs, some still run by volunteer organizations, many now integrated into municipal garbage collection systems.

Among the earliest recycling efforts were the bottle bills of the 1960s, when legislation was introduced in many states mandating a five-to-ten-cent deposit return on bottles and cans. These bills were a response to the litter problem along American highways. One study of the time reported that a representative mile of American highway was likely to turn up 710 beer cans, 143 soft drink cans, and 227 bottles and jars. The bottle bills were promoted as reducing litter, saving energy and natural resources, and reducing the volume of municipal waste.[13]

It has been estimated that if all the household recycling programs were to be perfectly efficient, they could lead to a reduction in municipal waste on the order of 24 percent. Unfortunately, efficiencies are nowhere near perfect, and current recovery rates in the United States run about 7 percent.[14] In the first place, only a small percent of all communities have recycling programs, and even in those communities that have them, not all citizens participate. There is also the long-standing problem of improper household sorting. One study found that 15 percent of the material put out in blue boxes for recycling was in fact nonrecyclable.[15]

The real problems, however, are economic. The political acceptance of government-run recycling programs has almost always been tied to a no-net-cost policy. Municipalities have repeatedly promised their constituents that all the costs of collection would be offset by the sale of the recyclable material. Unfortunately, the sale of recyclables has not always gone smoothly. In the commercial sector, the recycling business has been rife with failures over the years. Supply often outstrips demand, and prices fall too low to keep the recycling centers solvent. Programs run by municipal governments fall prey to the same market swings and cannot always meet the no-net-cost promises. A more realistic view is that recycling of household garbage must be recognized as something societally desirable, and like all desirable things it is likely to have a cost. As William Rathje and Cullen Murphy conclude in their offbeat and informative book *Rubbish! The Archeology of Garbage*, "Recycling is a fragile and complicated piece of economic and social machinery—a space shuttle rather than a tractor; it may break down frequently." They warn against a misdirected search for a garbage panacea that "conserves resources, turns a profit, and saves the world."[16]

Recycling of household municipal waste is an important component of any integrated waste-management strategy, but it is not a panacea. With current technologies and the current level of public support, the percentage of the total waste load that is realistically recyclable is small. Given current population projections, it is unlikely that the anticipated growth in recycling can even keep pace with the anticipated growth in the waste load in urban centers. Recycling is imperative and valuable, but its potential to reduce waste loads is limited, and putting an effective system in place is expensive and politically difficult. It is part of the solution, but not *the* solution.

The other side of the waste reduction equation is the recycling of hazardous industrial waste. Surprisingly, the considerable successes in this area have received very little press. The fact is when it comes to the protection of human health, reduction in the volume of industrial waste streams is of much greater import than the reduction in the volume of municipal waste. Of course, both strategies serve to reduce the demand for landfill and incinerator capacity, and in this sense they both have social value, but if we are trying to have a direct impact on the health of the nation, the greatest potential lies in the industrial sector.

Fortunately, there have been major strides in the past couple of decades in the recycling of industrial wastes. Table 13 lists some of the

Table 13 Recyclable wastes from certain industrial processes.

Industry	Recyclable Waste
Oil refining	wastewater, waste oil
Electroplating	copper, nickel, chromium
Paint	spray-gun sludge
Photo processing	silver, process chemicals
Textile	waste dye, wastewater, process chemicals
Printing	ink, solvents
Automobile	used lubricating oil
Dry cleaning	solvents

recyclable wastes associated with several industrial processes.[17] These materials include metals, solvents, and waste oils, all of which figured prominently in my earlier discussion of chemicals of environmental concern.

The economics of waste reduction and recycling in the industrial sector are often more favorable than in the municipal sector. The increasing price over the years of petroleum products and solvents, the decreasing costs of recycling systems, and the increasing costs of disposal brought about by the Superfund and RCRA regulations have all served to make it more cost-effective to eliminate waste and promote reuse. The economics of industrial recycling are likely to improve even further in future years. In recent years, many companies have set up special divisions to research new markets for their by-products and recycled waste. The Surplus Products Group of Union Carbide, for example, has been turning a profit for many years.[18] To quote one observer of the chemical industry, "In many ways, the rogue's gallery of the worst polluters of the 1960s are becoming the corporate environmentalists of the 1990s."[19]

Undoubted strides have been taken, but as with municipal recycling activities, current industrial recycling activity is nowhere near its full potential. It has been estimated, for example, that 80 percent of used lubricating oil could be recycled; current efforts run around 10 percent.[20]

However, as with the municipal sector, even if some of this potential were realized, we would still be hard-pressed to keep up with the pace of industrial growth. Industrial recycling is an important part of our national waste-management strategy, but like household recycling, it cannot be viewed as a cure-all. It will not negate the need for the siting of new industrial landfills and the development of increased incineration capacity for industrial wastes.

There is also the sad fact that not all recycling activities are themselves benign. The recycling of newspaper, for example, generates hazardous chemical waste from the de-inking process. One of the saddest cases on the Superfund ledger is the Western Processing site near Seattle, Washington. It was a recycling center to end all recycling centers: battery acid recovery, transformer fluid recovery, solvent recycling, tire storage, gasohol generation. If it was in the recycling lexicon, Western Processing was in the business. The owner of the site was a one-man entrepreneur of the environmental occult. He was in the recycling game long before it became politically correct. Sadly, while his heart was in the right place, his waste control practices were not, and the site became one of the more notorious Superfund sites in the state. As a general observation, an Office of Technology Assessment study commented that "it is not always clear whether secondary manufacturing produces less pollution per ton of material processed than primary manufacturing."[21]

And of course there are some wastes that just seem to resist the very idea of being recycled. Americans throw out more than 200 million tires a year, and most of them remain in huge piles at selected dumps across the nation. Every once in a while, one of these piles catches fire and hits the front pages of your newspaper. Many recycling schemes have been proposed and tried, but nothing yet tried has proven to be sufficiently profitable. Of course, it must be noted that many environmentalists claim that the problem lies not in the profitability of the recycling schemes but in the profitability of the primary industries, whose leaders systematically oppose and discourage recycling initiatives in the belief that their bottom lines will ultimately suffer.

Enough on the downside; let's end this section on a high note. Most people are not aware that it is possible to generate energy from landfills.

Most municipal landfills generate gases, primarily methane, and at many landfills these gases are being captured and used to produce energy. At the Keele Valley landfill in Toronto, methane production drives a 30-megawatt electrical generating plant. In the United States, the EPA has estimated that landfill gases could produce energy equivalent to the output from 400,000 barrels of oil per day, enough to satisfy the nation's commercial and residential lighting needs. Unfortunately, to date only 1 percent of this energy has been harnessed. In Denmark, Switzerland, Sweden, and the Netherlands, the recovery rate is closer to 30 percent.[22]

Apart from the energy conservation aspect, there is a further environmental benefit to the recovery of landfill gases. Landfills currently release 30–70 million tons of methane per year into the atmosphere, 16–18 percent of the total methane released worldwide. Methane is a so-called "greenhouse gas." It has a more severe effect on the atmosphere than carbon dioxide. The capture of landfill gases thus has a role to play in the prevention of global warming.

So, is recycling the answer? In a word, no. Is recycling an important and valuable component in the mix of waste-management strategies needed to keep our waste problems under control? Of course. We should support it and improve it. But we shouldn't lose our perspective: it is not a panacea.

LANDFILLS FOREVER, OR SOMETHING LIKE THEM

With the ever-increasing volumes of solid municipal waste and hazardous industrial waste, and recognizing the realistic limitations of recovery and recycling, we are left with a Hobson's choice: incineration or landfilling. One pollutes the air, the other pollutes the land and water. It seems inescapable that we will see lots of both technologies well into the foreseeable future.

Our interest here centers on the landfilling option. How bad is it? Are there ways that we might reduce the environmental impact?

Historically, the first "sanitary" landfills were developed in the

1920s.[23] The fact that they are now considered a major environmental problem is somewhat ironic in that they were originally developed to replace foul-smelling open dumps and reduce the need for uncontrolled incineration. By the 1960s, of course, it had become clear that the containment capabilities of these early landfills were inadequate to prevent groundwater contamination. One study has estimated that 75 percent of the 75,000 municipal and industrial landfills in the United States are leaking.[24] Another identified 27 cases of groundwater pollution in 385 site-years of operation at 39 hazardous-waste landfills, a failure rate of 69 percent.[25] Public alarm over such statistics led legislators and regulatory agencies in either of two directions. They either tried to clamp down on the number of new landfills, or they tried to enforce more stringent specifications on landfill design.

The most extreme version of the first approach took the form of an outright ban on all landfilling of hazardous waste. Such a law was first passed in California in 1981. At the federal level, the Hazardous and Solid Waste Amendments to RCRA, enacted in 1984, identified land disposal as the "least favorable" approach to waste disposal. It was argued that landfilling should be retained only for residues remaining after "effective hazardous waste treatment." Both these programs were expected to encourage a massive increase in treatment plant capacity for hazardous wastes. Unfortunately, this anticipated growth never came to pass. It turns out that public fear of treatment facilities runs almost as high as for landfills. Proposed treatment projects were frustrated by difficulties in siting, fear of intrusive regulatory control, and economic uncertainties. In addition, many waste-generating firms found it cheaper to dispose of their wastes in old landfills that were still operating under grandfather clauses in the new regulations, rather than to engage the services of the new (and expensive) waste-treatment firms. As these old landfills began to close, waste generators were left holding the bag: no new landfills, and no new treatment plants. The main impact of the landfill-ban bills turned out to be an unintended one: a severe shortage of hazardous-waste-disposal capacity.

At the same time, environmentalists and government regulators began to realize that treatment is not necessarily more environmentally benign than landfilling. In recent years, landfills have become more respectable again, but only if they conform to the very strict new specifications for design and construction. All major landfills constructed under RCRA rules since about 1990 must have basal liners, protective covers, and gas and leachate collection systems.[26] Some basal liners consist of compacted clay, but most are synthetic geomembranes of high-density polyethylene (HDPE). The most recent EPA regulations require the use of these impermeable synthetic membranes. As mentioned in chapter 2, it is now usual to have more than one liner, separated by properly designed drainage layers that are integrated with a carefully designed leachate collection system. As of 1991, the EPA requires "six layers of protection" between the waste and the underlying groundwater. The engineering design objective of this approach would appear to be "entombment forever."

However, this line of thinking is severely flawed. The "failure" of a landfill occurs when there is a release of contaminated leachate due to a breach in the containment system. Failures may occur under any of the scenarios described in chapter 2. They may occur early in the life of the landfill due to poor engineering design and construction, or they may occur during the operational stage due to human error. But even if careful quality control eliminates these types of failures (and nowadays it is hopefully only in the rarest of cases that such failures would occur), landfills are still prone to the "longevity catch." There is no getting around the fact that liners, covers, and leachate collection systems cannot last forever. They have a finite life expectancy, and at some point in the future even the most well-constructed landfill will begin to leak. There is much controversy over how long a landfill liner can be expected to function, but the most defensible estimates probably lie in the range of 50 to 100 years. After that time, contamination of the surrounding environment will commence. Current design methodologies that emphasize engineered entombment do not satisfy the basic tenet of a defensible environmental ethic; they do not prevent the passing on of environmental risk to future generations. The engineering community has much to explain for its continued reliance on this flawed design framework.

One defense that the engineering community offers is the possibility of improved leachate quality over time. Given the delay time provided by entombment, is there perhaps hope that landfill leachates might lose their kick before they begin to escape into the environment? There have been many studies of the chemical quality of landfill leachates over time. Over the short periods of record available to date, there is not much hard evidence to suggest that leachates become more benign with time. However, in theory, over the long term, as the biodegradation process proceeds inside the landfill, one would anticipate reductions in the chemical concentrations of organic contaminants. Some researchers claim that leachates could become harmless within about 200 years.[27] There is a lot of uncertainty associated with these estimates, and in any case it is an open question as to whether landfill liners can be expected to last anywhere near this long, but perhaps this line of reasoning offers some solace. These estimates don't address the question of the heavy metals, however, which are not biodegraded and which will continue to be leached out of the landfill forever.

With respect to organic chemicals, which are the most ubiquitous toxins in landfill leachate, the question of leachate quality revolves around the efficiency of the biodegradation process in the landfill. A landfill can be viewed as an "inelegant biological reactor,"[28] in which waste decomposes over time under the influence of microbial action. Most landfills that rely on entombment are "dry" landfills that favor aerobic biodegradation (i.e., degradation in the presence of oxygen). In recent years there has been a move toward "wet" landfill designs that promote both aerobic and anaerobic (i.e., without oxygen) degradation. The goal of "wet" landfills is to produce accelerated biodegradation that might render landfill leachates less toxic over a shorter time span. The idea first emerged in the 1960s, and has always been considered a maverick idea in traditional engineering circles. However, recent successes have brought more credibility. Wet landfilling is quite popular in many countries, including Canada, where the largest landfill in the country, the Keele Valley landfill, is operated under this concept. Wet landfills have not found favor in the United States, where federal guidance strongly encourages dry entombment. In fact, wet landfills are actually illegal in many states.

Finally, there is the question of long-term administrative control. Given that prevention of environmental degradation from new landfills will require effective performance for many decades (or perhaps even centuries) after the period of waste emplacement, it is reasonable to ask whether current corporate structures and current regulatory practice can achieve this long-term control. Society in general does not have a very encouraging record in keeping institutional controls in place over such long time periods.

In summary, there is some cause for cautious hope. It is certainly fair to say that new landfills, with their improved design specifications, are much less likely to leak than old landfills, at least over the short term. In the long term, it is possible, although not fully proven, that impacts may be less severe. Nevertheless, it must be recognized that landfills really just delay, attenuate, and possibly reduce groundwater pollution rather than prevent it forever.

This section has dealt almost exclusively with design. We have not yet looked at the issue of siting. Mightn't it be possible through judicious siting of landfills (and other waste-management facilities) to reduce the impact of their apparently unavoidable long-term failure? In order to address this question, we must first look more carefully at the processes that lead to the migration of contaminants in the subsurface.

OUT OF SIGHT BUT NOT OUT OF MIND: WHAT HAPPENS TO CONTAMINANTS IN THE SUBSURFACE

By now it should be clear that there are a countless number of scenarios that can lead to the release of toxic chemicals into the environment. Releases arise from human carelessness, from poor engineering design, from inadequate operational procedures, and sometimes perhaps from malicious intent. In the past they have occurred most often from old waste-management facilities that were designed without containment capabilities, and from newer facilities with containment systems that were left in place longer than their design life. The result is landfill leachates, pipeline losses, and leaking underground tanks. I have de-scribed in some detail these different sources of contamination and the types of chemicals they are likely to release. What I have not done as yet is discuss what happens to these chemicals after their release. We must look more closely at what the EPA calls the "fate and transport" of these chemicals in the environment.

If someone were to dump a fifty-five-gallon drum of the solvent TCE in the back forty, where would it end up? How likely is it that this carcinogenic chemical would wind up in our drinking-water supply at concentrations harmful to our health? To answer these questions, we must look at the processes that control the migration of fluids through porous media. The fluids in question are air, water, and pure-phase TCE. The porous media in question are the soils and rocks that make up the shallow geologic environment into which the chemicals are released.

Understanding the processes of fate and transport is the first step in making predictions of the rates and distances of migration of contami-nants in the subsurface environment.[29] Predictions are usually carried out with simplified models of the processes, and these models require estimates of the parameter values used to quantify the processes. There is often a great deal of uncertainty in the values that should be assigned to these parameters, and this leads to considerable uncertainty in the quantitative predictions of fate and transport. The processes themselves, however, are relatively well understood. So let us begin there.

For the purposes of discussion, let us consider a site with very simple geology: a layer of sand twenty feet thick overlying bedrock of fractured shale. Let us assume further that the water table is at a depth of ten feet, so that all of the fractures in the shale, and all of the intergranular pores in the bottom half of the sand, are filled with water, whereas the pores in the upper ten feet of the sand are only partially filled with water. We refer to the zone below the water table as the saturated zone and the water therein as groundwater. We refer to the zone above the water table as the unsaturated zone and the water therein as soil water. In the un-saturated zone, those portions of the soil pores not filled with water contain air.

Now comes the careless release of a spilled drum of TCE onto the ground surface. The TCE enters the unsaturated zone and begins to move downward under gravity, thus introducing a third fluid into the system to go along with the air and water already present. The fate and transport of the TCE in the unsaturated zone is controlled by five processes: residualization, volatilization, dissolution, sorption, and biodegradation. The first of these processes is physical; the next three are chemical; and the last is biological. We will look at each briefly in turn.

Under the residualization process, some of the TCE is immobilized in the unsaturated zone and prevented from migrating downward to the water table. This immobilized TCE is held under tension between the sand grains, in the same way that the soil water is held. The fraction of the original spill that continues to move toward the water table as free product depends on the physical properties of the TCE (its density and viscosity), the properties of the porous media through which it is flowing (its porosity and permeability), and the depth to the water table.

The density of a fluid is a measure of its mass per unit volume. Water has a density of one gram per milliliter (g/mL), or one kilogram per liter (kg/L). Air is less dense than water and has a density much less than one. Most solvents, including TCE, are more dense than water and have densities greater than one. The viscosity of a fluid is a measure of its frictional resistance to flow. Water has a low viscosity; many waste oils have a high viscosity. Direct migration of free-product contaminant to the water table is enhanced by higher densities and lower viscosities. The solvent chloroform has higher density and lower viscosity than TCE. If our hypothetical spill were chloroform rather than TCE, it would migrate more effectively to the water table, with less residualization.

The two properties of the porous media that control flow are the porosity and the permeability. They are often confused, but they are conceptually quite separable. Porosity is a *storage* parameter; permeability is a *transmission* parameter. Porosity is a measure of the percentage of pore space in a soil or rock. The porosity of sand is often around 30 percent. In most fractured rocks, the only pore spaces that contribute to flow are the fractures themselves, so porosities are usually much lower. In highly fractured rock, porosities may run as high as 5 percent; but in sparsely fractured rock, porosities may be as small as 0.01 percent. The porosity controls the amount of space available for the residence of sub-surface fluids. For our spilled drum of TCE, higher porosity would promote greater residualization; lower porosity would promote greater delivery of free-product TCE to the water table.

Permeability is the property that controls the rate of transmission of fluids through porous media. It is strongly influenced by porosity (hence the confusion), but it also reflects the structure and fabric of the soil or rock. Sand and gravel have high permeability, leading to rapid rates of fluid migration. Clays have low permeability and slow rates of fluid migration. Most fractured rocks are of lower permeability (although there are exceptions, such as cavernous limestones and some types of volcanic rocks). For our TCE spill, the high-permeability sand postulated in our example would promote rapid migration of free-product TCE to the water table.

Unfortunately, even if the TCE were completely residualized in the unsaturated zone, this would not imply that none of the chemical would ever reach the water table. To see why, we must turn to the chemical processes in our original list. First of all, there are two chemical partitioning processes that have the potential to redistribute TCE mass between the three fluid phases. There may be volatilization of TCE into the soil air, and there may be dissolution of TCE into the soil water. Both the air phase and the water phase may themselves be mobile, leading to additional fluid motion that can spread the contaminant mass throughout the unsaturated zone in the vicinity of the spill. The circulation pattern of the soil air is usually directed back to the ground surface, leading to releases of volatilized TCE gas into the atmosphere. The circulation pattern of the soil water is usually directed downward toward the water table, leading to delivery of dissolved TCE to the groundwater.

There are two additional processes that may affect the mass of dissolved TCE delivered to the water table. The first is sorption, whereby some portion of the TCE becomes sorbed onto the soil particles. Sorption is enhanced by the presence of organic carbon in the soil and discouraged by its absence. The second is biodegradation, whereby some of the TCE is removed from the system as a nutrient for microorganisms living in the soil. Both these processes tend to reduce the mass of TCE moving downward through the unsaturated zone.

The degree of chemical partitioning of a contaminant between free product, soil air, soil water, sorbed mass, and bionutrient is controlled by the properties of the chemical, the properties of the soil, and the nature of the microorganic populations. The properties of the chemical that control its fate and transport are: (1) its solubility, which controls the dissolution process; (2) its air/water partition coefficient, which controls the volatilization process; (3) its soil/water partition coefficient, which controls the sorption process; and (4) its half-life, which describes the rate of the biodegradation process. Table 14 provides a summary of the likelihood of each of these processes being important for some of the chemicals identified earlier as being of environmental concern.[30] The differences between chemicals can be quite striking. For example, the solvent methylene chloride (MC) has very high solubility (13,200 mg/L) and low sorptive capacity, suggesting that this contaminant is likely to exhibit high concentrations in groundwater and that it can be very mobile. The wood-preserving chemical pentachlorophenol (PCP), on the other hand, is only sparingly soluble (14 mg/L) and is strongly sorbed, suggesting a low-concentration, immobile contaminant. Those contaminants in Table 14 that exhibit high volatility are likely to lose a goodly portion of their mass to the soil air and thence to the atmosphere. Those contaminants with high sorptive capacity will lose much of their mass as sorption onto organic matter in the near-surface soils. Biodegradation is most effective for petroleum hydrocarbons (the BTEX chemicals: benzene, toluene, ethylene, and xylene); it is less effective for the solvents.

A NAPL A DAY:
SOURCES, SOURCE AREAS, AND PLUMES

So what happens to this contaminant mass after it reaches the water table? Following the arguments of the previous section, it may arrive in one of three forms: as the chemical itself (the so-called free product), dissolved in infiltrating soil water, or volatilized in the circulating soil air. At most sites by far the greatest amount of mass arrives by the first of these three routes: direct migration of the free product. It has become common in technical circles to refer to this free product as *non-aqueous-*

Table 14 Fate and transport of selected chemicals.

Class	Chemical	Density*	Solubility	Volatility	Sorptive Capacity	Biodegradation Potential
Petroleum hydrocarbons	Benzene	L	Low	High	Moderate	High
Solvents	TCE	D	Moderate	High	Moderate	Low
	PCE	D	Low	High	Moderate	Low
	MC	D	Very high	Moderate	Low	Low
	CTC	D	Low	High	Moderate	Low
	VC	L	Very low	High	Low	Low
Wood-preserving chemicals	PCP	D	Very low	Very low	High	Low
PCBs	PCB	D	Moderate	Low	High	Moderate
Pesticides	EDB	D	Moderate	Low	High	Moderate
	Chlordane	D	Low	Low	High	Moderate

*L = LNAPL; D = DNAPL (see next section).

phase liquid, which simply means that it is a liquid that is not water. This terminology has led to the wide usage of the acronym NAPL, which has a faintly ridiculous sound to it, but which has come to strike fear into the hearts of owners of contaminated sites. As we shall see in chapter 5, the presence of a NAPL at a contaminated site has important ramifications with respect to the feasibility of site remediation.

Non-aqueous-phase liquids are further classified as LNAPL (L for "light"; pronounced *el-napple*) and DNAPL (D for "dense"; pronounced *dee-napple*). It is an important distinction for fate and transport, and for remediation. LNAPLs are less dense than water, and they float on the water table. DNAPLs are denser than water, and they sink through the water table into the underlying groundwater. If we think back to the "contaminants that matter," in Table 3, most petroleum hydrocarbons (oil and gasoline) are LNAPLs, while most solvents, wood-preserving chemicals, PCBs, and pesticides are DNAPLs. If we think back to the Ville Mercier case history introduced in chapter 1, this is exactly how these fluids layered themselves in the waste lagoon at that site. The BTEX chemicals (benzene, toluene, ethylene, and xylene) floated on the surface of the lagoon. The wood preservatives and solvents sank to the base. The LNAPLs are *floaters* and the DNAPLs are *sinkers*. The same distinction holds true at the water table.

Once in the saturated zone below the water table, the DNAPLs continue to residualize just as they did in the unsaturated zone above the water table. They become trapped and immobilized in pools, blobs, and stringy ganglia of free product within the pores and fractures of the soil or rock. Their downward mobility is impeded by layers and lenses of low-permeability materials. At most sites that have been fully investigated, there is usually some depth below which DNAPLs are no longer encountered.

The anatomy of a contaminated site can be viewed as having three elements: (1) the *source*, which is the landfill, waste lagoon, spill, or leak that gives rise to the site; (2) the *source area*, which is the extended region in the vicinity of the source that encompasses all the residualized pools of LNAPLs and DNAPLs; and (3) the dissolved contaminant *plume* that emanates from the source area.[31]

We usually don't think of oil and gas (or solvents, for that matter) as being soluble in water. We are taught in grade school that "oil and water don't mix," and in the main this is true. Oil and water (and solvents and water) are immiscible fluids that retain their separate phases, even if one tries to mix them. However, while oil and solvents don't mix readily with water, they are not totally insoluble. The solubilities, while low, are large enough to create dissolved plumes in groundwater, with contaminant concentrations that far exceed the established health standards. These dissolved contaminant plumes take the form of long skinny snakes of contaminated water that originate in the source area and then slowly migrate downstream with the flowing groundwater.

In order to put us all on the same page, it is necessary to digress for a moment and consider the characteristics of naturally occurring groundwater flow systems.[32] Many people have an image of subsurface water flow as an "underground river," but this is an inaccurate and misleading conceptual model. While an "underground river," or something like it, may occur in a limestone cave (which is, I suppose, the only place where most people ever actually see groundwater), it is far from the norm. A much better conceptual model is that of a large sponge, sitting on a sloping table, with water dripping in at the top end and dripping out at the bottom end. The sponge represents the geological environment. All the pores are filled with water, and the water is slowly oozing through all the pores of the sponge, from the top of the slope toward the bottom.

In real hydrogeological environments, flow systems develop that deliver groundwater flow from recharge areas in the highlands to discharge areas in the valleys. Recharge occurs from rainfall and snowmelt; discharge occurs as evapotranspiration from valley bottoms and as base flow to streams. The flow system is strongly influenced by the geological materials through which the flow passes. One usually differentiates between aquifers, which are high-permeability geologic formations in which flow is fast, and aquitards, which are low-permeability geologic formations in which flow is slow. The terms "fast" and "slow" are relative: even the fastest groundwater flow in the most permeable aquifers is really quite slow, no more than a few tens to a few hundred feet per year.

Figure 10 shows a contaminant plume (in plan and in cross-section) from the Otis Air Force Base on Cape Cod, Massachusetts.[33] The hydrogeological environment at this site is very similar to the hypothetical case I described earlier: high-permeability sand over low-permeability clay with a shallow water table. The contaminant plume that emerges from the source area (some "filter beds" used for liquid waste disposal) is a long, skinny snake that flows downstream in the direction of regional groundwater flow within the saturated zone of the sand aquifer.

The process by which dissolved contamination is carried away from source areas by flowing groundwater is known as advective transport. The rates of advective transport have been carefully measured for advancing contaminant plumes at two field research sites, the U.S. Geological Survey site at the Otis Air Force Base described above and a site studied by the University of Waterloo at the Borden Air Force Base in Ontario.[34] (The use of air force bases in both cases is not totally coincidental: such bases are notorious for carelessness in their past solvent usage during airplane degreasing and are the settings for many well-known plumes.) The measured rates of plume-front migration at the two sites were 250 and 60 feet per year, respectively. At two of the longest Superfund plumes, one near Tucson, Arizona, and the other in the San Fernando Valley, California, both over five miles long, back calculations relating the distance traveled by the plumes to the assumed dates of source initiation indicate advective transport rates on the order of 500 feet per year.

While advection is the primary process of contaminant migration in the saturated zone, many of the same secondary processes that occur in the unsaturated zone are also at work here. In particular, sorption of solvents onto organic matter in the aquifer and biodegradation of petroleum hydrocarbons can remove mass from the advancing plume, reducing concentrations and retarding the rate of advance of the plume front relative to the rate of flowing groundwater. For some chemicals in some aquifers, the degree of retardation can be significant, reaching factors of ten, one hundred, or even more for particularly sorptive chemicals.

Not much has been said about metals here, or radionuclides. As I noted earlier these chemical species may be just as toxic (or even more so) than the organic contaminants. Their fate and transport, however, is

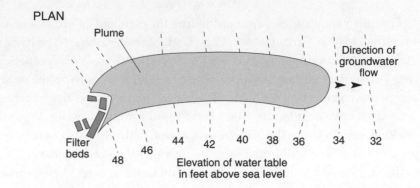

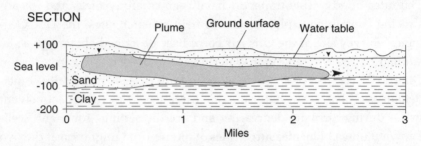

Figure 10. Plume of groundwater contamination at Otis Air Force Base, Cape Cod, Massachusetts. (After D. R. Leblanc, ed., *Movement and Fate of Solutes in a Plume of Sewage Contaminated Groundwater, Cape Cod, Massachusetts,* U.S. Geological Survey Open File Report 84-475 [Washington, D.C.: U.S. Government Printing Office, 1984].)

much simpler. They do not residualize, or volatilize, or form LNAPLs or DNAPLs. They move through the subsurface system (both unsaturated and saturated) in dissolved form via advective transport. They can be strongly retarded due to sorption, in some cases almost to the point of immobility. There is some evidence that microbial action can influence their transport, but the level of research understanding in this area is still emerging.

So, if we return to that spilled drum of TCE (or for that matter, to a stringer of contaminated leachate emerging from the base of a failed landfill), it is now clear that these liquids enter a complex physical-chemical-hydrogeological system, with many interacting processes at work. However, the dominant process at most sites, and the one that matters most in terms of aquifer contamination, is the simple advective transport provided by flowing groundwater. As we return to the siting issue, this is where my discussion will begin.

THE TECHNICAL IMPORTANCE OF SITING

The first thing to note from the previous section is that at all of the contaminated sites mentioned there (Cape Cod, Mass.; Borden, Ontario; Tucson, Ariz.; and San Fernando, Calif.), as well as at many of the other sites mentioned earlier (Hanford, Wash.; Rocky Flats, Colo.; Woburn, Mass.; and Toms River, N.J.), the dissolved contaminant plume is migrating through a shallow, surficial, high-permeability sand-and-gravel aquifer, similar to the conditions I postulated for the hypothetical TCE spill. It is worth asking whether groundwater contamination ever occurs in any other type of hydrogeological environment.

The rate of flow in any particular geologic horizon can be estimated using Darcy's Law, named after the nineteenth-century French hydraulic engineer Henry Darcy, who first developed it and recognized its importance as one of the basic, empirical laws of physics. (And yes, his first name was Henry, not Henri.) Darcy's law states that the advective flow velocity in porous media is a function of the permeability of the porous media and the hydraulic gradient of the flow system. For near-surface flow systems, the kind that are of most interest in contaminant transport studies, one can think of the hydraulic gradient as being controlled by the slope of the water table, which in turn often mirrors the topographic slope of the land.

Permeability can vary over many orders of magnitude between different soil and rock types, and Darcy's Law tells us that the rate of groundwater flow is linearly related to the permeability of the aquifer through which it moves. In other words, if the aquifer permeability were two orders of magnitude smaller than the appropriate value for sand and gravel, as would be the case for, say, a silty sand, then the rates of advective transport would be reduced from hundreds of feet per year to a few feet per year. If the permeability were several orders of magnitude less, as would be the case for clays and shales, then the advective transport rates would be less than one foot per year. It is not surprising, then, that almost all the most notorious Superfund sites are sited on very-high-permeability aquifers, because it is only in this type of geologic formation that a plume is likely to advance sufficiently far from its source area to come to public attention. While sand-and-gravel aquifers are perhaps the most common, there are other kinds of aquifers that can have permeabilities that are as high or higher. These include fractured sandstones, porous volcanic rocks, and karstic limestones (the type of limestones that host Carlsbad Caverns and Mammoth Caves). There are many contaminated sites in North America that are fortuitously situated on lower-permeability deposits and have therefore not created dissolved contaminant plumes that threaten our aquifers and drinking-water supplies. Many of these sites have not come to public attention, because in terms of public health, they just don't matter.

Clearly, this line of reasoning has strong implications with respect to the siting of future waste-management facilities, especially landfills, which we now know are almost bound to leak at some future date. If we could site these facilities on low-permeability terrain, we would be assured that contamination would not migrate to any great distance, perhaps for thousands of years. And what little migration does occur would not threaten drinking-water supplies, because low-permeability rocks and soils seldom constitute viable aquifers for the development of water supplies.

In one research study of alternative landfill sites in which a "failure" was defined as a breach of the containment structure followed by contaminant migration via advective groundwater flow to a compliance well, the probability of failure was shown to be reduced from 75 percent (failure in three out of four cases) for a high-permeability site, to 0.0005 percent (failure in 1 case in 200,000) for a low-permeability site.[35] In short, the effects of good siting on potential environmental degradation can be huge.

Of course, there *would* be contaminated source areas, replete with

LNAPLs and DNAPLs, in the vicinity of the facilities in due course, after the breakdown of the containment system, but these would be local. Such a situation is infinitely preferable to the ubiquitous presence of contaminated plumes snaking through our water-supply aquifers. If it is possible to maintain proper public records of all decommissioned waste-management facilities without loss of administrative control, it should be possible to protect the public from direct contact with contaminants in the source areas through surface control measures (warning signs, fencing, capping, etc.). While it is true that past experience does not provide much encouragement for the likely success of long-term administrative control of such sites, perhaps special efforts could be put forth to try to improve societal performance in this arena. Certainly, the task of surface control is a more feasible, more cost-effective approach to human-health protection than trying to control subsurface contaminant plumes.

Legislators and regulators have been loathe to enter the siting fray. The RCRA regulations, for example, discuss the design specifications for the six layers of protection in great detail, but provide only vague guidance with respect to siting. One type of regulatory program that *does* bear on this issue is the wellhead protection programs that have been instituted in some jurisdictions. These programs do not specify where waste-management facilities should be sited, but rather where they should *not* be sited, namely, within the capture zones of major water supply wells. Some programs have gone even further by disallowing such facilities over entire watersheds or over the recharge areas of major aquifers. These programs represent a form of zoning, which is a traditional government prerogative of long standing. One might well ask why these zoning powers cannot be brought to bear in the specification of acceptable waste-management sites as well as unacceptable ones.

Some environmental writers go even further. They suggest that because really favorable sites are so few and far between, we should consider establishing national hazardous-waste-management sites (much as is being proposed for high-level nuclear waste) at a few of the very best sites.[36] An initial candidate area in western South Dakota has even been proposed.[37]

The arguments in favor of careful siting seem so clear that it is reasonable to ask why we have not moved farther in this direction. After all, when past design practices were found wanting, regulators leaped in with tighter specifications. Now that past siting practices have been similarly exposed (witness, for example, the use of the abandoned gravel pit at Ville Mercier, probably the worst site that could conceivably have been selected), why aren't regulators taking a similarly proactive stand? The answer lies in our participatory, democratic style of government and its sometimes seamy companion, politics. In the province of Ontario, for example, the provincial government created the Ontario Waste Management Corporation (OWMC) for the sole purpose of siting and constructing a hazardous-waste facility. The corporation carried out a technical siting program, investigating hundreds of sites across the province, then gradually narrowing things down to a few of the best sites that were selected for intensive investigation. There was little reaction from the public until one site was actually selected, then a public uproar ensued. The government backed off and no site was ever selected under the OWMC program.

It seems unfortunate, but having identified proper technical siting of waste-management facilities as the feature that offers us the most hope for environmental protection, it turns out to be the one that founders first on our proud democratic tradition. We have entered the world of NIMBY (Not In My Back Yard), and like Alice at the Mad Hatter's tea party, it is hard to see how to escape.

THE SOCIAL DIFFICULTIES OF SITING

We tend to think of the NIMBY syndrome as something modern, an outgrowth of our more participatory democracy and the current chic for public protest. It may come as a surprise then to read the following words, written by the chief health officer of Washington, D.C., in 1889: "Appropriate places for garbage are becoming scarcer year by year. . . . Already the inhabitants in proximity to the public dumps are beginning to complain."[38]

The NIMBY syndrome is a true "tragedy of the commons,"[39] in which policies that benefit the community at large, such as the siting of regional waste-management facilities, may not benefit all the individuals in that community, and may indeed bring costs and risks to some that exceed the benefits. It is not unreasonable for people who are put in such a position to believe that they are being asked to unfairly shoulder the burden of others, and to seek redress from this unfair burden.

The thing that is new about the current spate of NIMBY-based protests is the degree to which they are succeeding. In recent years, under the influence of NIMBY protest, there has been a precipitous decline in both the number of operating landfills and in the number of new landfill sites approved and permitted for construction. In New Jersey, for example, the number of operating landfills has declined from 300 to 15 in recent years.[40] In the nation as a whole, only 7 new hazardous-waste facilities were permitted and built between 1980 and 1986.[41] New York City had 89 landfills in 1934; by 1991 only 1 remained in operation.[42]

The single remaining landfill in New York City is the huge Fresh Kills landfill discussed earlier, but despite its massive size, it can accept only 10,000 of the 27,000 tons of garbage generated each day in the city.[43] The rest is shipped to Illinois. Worse yet, Fresh Kills is scheduled to close in the year 2005, and this is going to precipitate a true garbage crisis in the largest city in America. Constraints on air pollution militate against the construction of incinerators; recycling diverts only a small fraction of the waste that is generated; and NIMBY pressures block all attempts to site new landfills.

The success of NIMBY pressures may relate in part to the large number of stakeholders involved in the siting of a waste-management facility.[44] These include *responsible stakeholders*, such as the waste-management firm that owns the site, the waste generators who hope to use the facility, and the insurance company who holds the insurance policy for the waste-management firm; *regulatory stakeholders*, in the form of state and federal agencies such as the EPA; potentially *injured stakeholders* in the host community who fear health impacts and reduced property values; and *peripheral stakeholders* representing special interest groups like developers, farmers, sporting groups, labor unions, and environmental groups. Some of these stakeholders are affected by the problem, which in this case is inadequate waste-management capacity; others are affected by the solution, namely, the new facility. Some are affected directly, some indirectly; some beneficially, some adversely. In some cases, the perceived impacts are solely due to proximity. In other cases, the perceived impacts are sociopolitical, perhaps reflecting environmental values or attitudes toward government planning and regulation. No matter what the mix of stakeholders, it is almost always the case that the costs, benefits, and risks for the proposed facility are perceived differently by the different stakeholders. There is almost always an adversarial relationship, and very often the preferences of the various groups are simply incompatible.

The inability of our current political framework to successfully site needed waste-management facilities has strong societal implications. It encourages unacceptable waste-management practices, including the continued use of old, poorly designed, leaking landfills and the growth of illegal dumping. Such practices expose the public to much larger health risks than would accrue from properly designed modern facilities. In addition, it drives the waste-generating industries to relocate to friendlier jurisdictions, leading to a loss of jobs and a decline in economic health.

Land use decisions have traditionally been the prerogative of local governments, but when it comes to the siting of regional waste-management facilities, every state in the union and most provinces in Canada have recognized the need for higher-level intervention. Because local governments are subdivisions of state government, it has been possible for state governments to enact legislation to try to bring local governments into line with regional or state waste-management plans.[45] The methods that have been tried to impose this will can be classified as power-broking, negotiation, compensation, and tendering.[46]

Power-broking is the use of top-down, preemptive authority, without significant negotiation or public participation. A few states (including New Jersey and Minnesota, for example) have tried to use their full state power in the selection and authorization of waste-management sites, but the approach has rarely succeeded. This top-down approach leads to the four Rs: regulation, resentment, resistance, and refusal.[47] The result is usually public protest, litigation, and ultimately, political capitulation.

Negotiation has a more cooperative sound to it, but most states that use negotiated siting procedures (among them, California, Massachusetts, and Texas) reserve the right to override local decisions designed to block the proposed facilities. With these types of provisos in place, negotiation has not proven any more successful than power-broking.

The idea that offsetting compensation can be used to bribe host communities into accepting unwanted facilities has long been in vogue among environmental economists. Compensation can take the form of direct payments to local governments, tax incentives for the citizens of host communities, preferential hiring and purchasing in the host community, or regional developmental assistance. Despite the apparent logic of the idea, there is little evidence that economic incentives produce successful siting.[48] In one study, based on questionnaires completed by citizens of a potential host community, it was found that less than 10 percent of those originally opposed to the facility changed their mind when economic incentives were added to the package. These results probably reflect the fact that opposition to waste-management facilities is not solely economic.[49] Among the noneconomic issues that may dominate are the stigma of having a waste site in one's community, the loss of community control over land use, the perceived unfairness of the imposed burden, lack of confidence in regulatory agencies, and overriding all, the fear of health impacts. In the questionnaire-based study just mentioned, the addition of risk-mitigation proposals, such as more frequent safety inspections and improved spill-prevention programs, had greater impact in garnering support for the facility than did the economic incentives (although these proposals only changed the minds of 22 percent of those originally opposed). The general conclusion seems to be that support for unpopular facilities cannot be bought at any price.

The only siting approach with any real success to report is tendering, which includes a strong compensation component, but with a greater emphasis on public participation and the identification of willing host communities. In the tendering approach, state agencies announce that they are open to bids from potential host communities, on the understanding that the agency will accept the lowest-cost bid for facility siting. The "bids" take the form of demands for compensation, which may take any of the forms noted above, and demands for insurance against failure, which may include both technical assurance and a compensatory component.

The most widely reputed case history of a successful tendering process is the Alberta Special Waste Management Facility at Swan Hills, Alberta.[50] This is a fully integrated hazardous-waste treatment and disposal facility that can handle a complete spectrum of organic and inorganic waste. It was opened in 1987 following a tendering process in which five communities expressed an interest in hosting the facility. In the Alberta system, it was necessary that a plebiscite be held in the community, with an outcome that clearly supported the facility. In the community that ranked highest of the five applicants, this plebiscite failed, but in Swan Hills, which was the second choice, it passed handily. In one of the three communities not selected, disappointment ran so high that there were organized protests at the Alberta legislature over *not* being selected to host the facility. After ten years of operation the facility remains popular in the community; it provides more than ninety full-time jobs and is credited to a large degree for the economic stabilization of the town. However, there are still questions as to whether Swan Hills represents the best social decision for the citizens of Alberta. The site is located far from the urban centers of Calgary and Edmonton, where most of the hazardous waste is generated. Transportation costs are high, and there is public concern that much of the waste that ought to go to Swan Hills is not being directed there, for economic reasons.

In recent years, the need for grassroots public participation in waste-siting decisions has been more clearly recognized. It is certainly more in keeping with our democratic traditions, and one would think that the probability of site approval would be enhanced by a collaborative rather than a preemptive approach, one based on persuasion and negotiation rather than coercion. Most environmental handbooks also argue that the chances for success are improved by the wide dissemination of information to a diverse set of stakeholders, and by an open political process with well-publicized schedules and firm, clear contractual arrangements.

It would be nice to report that if such rules are followed, success is guaranteed, but this is not the case. There is no statistical evidence to suggest that the degree of success in facility siting has been appreciably changed by the greater levels of public participation. In recent years, siting successes have been few and far between, regardless of the approach taken. It is even possible as some have suggested that public participation is more likely to undermine decision-making than bring about harmony and consensus.[51] Even with public participation, NIMBY is alive and well and still awaiting the perfect solution.

The siting of waste-management facilities also raises ethical questions of equity and justice. A decision that is optimal in some sense for society as a whole will not be optimal for all of the individuals in the society. As Lester Thurow recognized in his concept of the "zero-sum society," there are always winners and losers associated with every social decision.[52] Host communities consist of many individuals who differ in their politics, values, and economic status. Some individuals are harmed by waste-management facilities; others stand to gain. Those with the lowest economic status generally have the least political power; and because there is a strong political component in the siting process, most waste-management facilities end up on the poor side of town. In short, those people who are least well-off are asked to shoulder the additional risks. If we view the purpose of social welfare schemes to be some measure of income redistribution, and if we recall the dollar-based definition of risk presented in chapter 2, then the current methods of siting waste-management facilities are not a part of the social welfare program.

Even the tendering approach can represent a Faustian bargain,[53] whereby waste-management companies offer to alleviate the economic woes of desperate communities through the siting of waste-management facilities. A cynic would not find it surprising that many of the poorer Indian reservations are offering to host such facilities, nor that waste-management companies are eager to accept, given that the reservations are not subject to state and federal environmental law.

One of the saddest cases of cultural conflict over the environment has occurred in Noxubee County, Mississippi,[54] where a hazardous-waste facility is under consideration. Wealthy whites oppose the facility and charge that the company trying to site the facility has chosen Noxubee County because of its concentration of poor and ill-educated blacks. Most blacks, on the other hand, support the project because it will provide jobs. The situation raises the specter of a kind of environmental racism that would not serve the nation well.

Even if politically acceptable procedures can be worked out, there is still the overriding question of how to integrate the technical needs of siting with the sociopolitical needs. As we saw at the end of the last section, the best technical site identified by the Ontario Waste Management Corporation turned out to be politically unacceptable. On the other hand, there is no guarantee that the sociopolitical procedures identified in this section will lead to the selection of sites that are technically suitable. I have discussed how favorable site hydrogeology can reduce the probability of failure of a waste-management facility (and hence the potential health risk to the public) by orders of magnitude. It seems imperative that site selection procedures pay heed to this reality.

Currently there are many potential sites that have reached gridlock at the technical/sociopolitical boundary. The low-level-radioactive-waste site at Ward Valley, California, sits in limbo under political opposition, even though the technical suitability of the site has been endorsed by a panel of seventeen experts assembled by the National Academy of Sciences.[55] (Although it must be admitted in this case that there were two dissenting opinions on the panel, and this has undoubtedly raised concern in many minds.) Even more peculiar is the case of the Waste Isolation Pilot Project. The WIPP is a subsurface repository for certain types of low-to-intermediate-level military nuclear waste that has already been constructed near Carlsbad, New Mexico, at a cost of hundreds of millions of dollars. The facility has the technical blessing of all reputable experts, yet it sat idle for years, prevented from serving its purpose by political wrangling. As pointed out by John B. Robertson, a hydrogeologist involved in the Ward Valley case, we seem to have entered a netherland where there are only two choices: "a licensed, operating site in a marginally acceptable hydrogeologic setting, or a site in the best possible hydrogeological setting that never opens for business."

At the present time, the siting problem remains unresolved. NIMBY groups continue to block needed projects at the local level. Higher-level

politicians put their heads in the sand and hope that contentious decisions can be postponed until after their term in office. Eventually, decisions will have to be made in crisis mode. It remains to be seen whether
such decisions will be able to honor both the technical needs of siting
and the sociopolitical realities.

THE SPECIAL CASE OF NUCLEAR WASTE

The technical and social issues associated with the siting of waste disposal facilities for municipal and industrial waste may appear daunting,
but they are like child's play when compared to the difficulties encountered in the search for a final resting place for the nation's high-level
nuclear waste. Many of the issues are the same in principle, but they are
multiplied a hundredfold by the public's fear and loathing of all things
nuclear. I will limit my discussion here to *high-level waste* (the spent fuel
rods from commercial nuclear reactors, and the liquid waste from the
military weapons programs), but most of the same issues apply to the
case of *low-level waste* (the less contaminated effluvia from the other
stages of the nuclear fuel cycle). In fact, when it comes to nuclear dread,
the public pays very little attention to words like "high-level" and "low-
level." It is the N-word that flips the switch, bringing images of Chernobyl and the apocalypse into clear focus.

There are about 430 commercial nuclear power plants worldwide, and
they produce about 17 percent of the world's electrical power.[56] In the
United States there are 107 reactors, almost all of them east of the Mississippi.[57] An average-size 1,000-megawatt nuclear power plant has
thousands of fuel rods in place at any given time. About one-third of
these are replaced annually, giving rise to a high-level-waste load of
about 30 tons of spent fuel per reactor per year. It is estimated that by
the year 2000 a total of 40,000 metric tons of high-level waste will have
been generated in the United States since the birth of the nuclear industry. This may sound like a lot, but on a volume basis it is far from over-
whelming. If it could be consolidated, it would all fit into a fifteen-foot-
high warehouse the size of a football field.[58]

None of this high-level waste has received permanent disposal. The spent fuel rods are currently stored in water-filled pools at the reactor sites. Surprisingly, they do not pose any additional threat to society in this form, over and above the threat posed by the presence of the reactor facilities themselves; but it is recognized in all the nuclear-power-generating nations of the world that some type of permanent disposal is needed.

In the United States, the beginning of the search for a permanent disposal site can be dated to 1957. Prior to that date, a variety of options were still under consideration, including shooting the waste into space and dumping it into deep ocean trenches.[59] However in 1957, a committee of the National Academy of Sciences recommended that future efforts be limited to consideration of a mined underground repository in a suitable geologic medium that would not allow the escape of radionuclides into the surface environment.[60] Initial efforts focused on deep salt beds because most salt formations are essentially free of fractures and they are known to have the lowest permeability of any naturally occurring rock type. An early attempt to utilize an abandoned salt mine in Kansas foundered on technical and social opposition, thus providing an early preview of all that has come to pass in the years since.

Bedded salt is the host rock for the only subsurface nuclear repository that has ever been built. It is the Waste Isolation Pilot Plant (the WIPP site) near Carlsbad, New Mexico, which began construction in 1979 as a permanent disposal site for the high-level liquid wastes generated by the U.S. military in its weapons programs. However, twenty years after the start of construction, and several years after its completion, the first nuclear waste was only just recently emplaced at the WIPP site. The facility was kept in constant readiness for years awaiting a resolution of the technopolitical storms that swirled around it.

Meanwhile, the civilian program has lurched along from crisis to crisis. The Nuclear Waste Policy Act of 1982 called for the investigation of multiple sites in different geological environments, and it mandated full public participation in the siting decision. It established the Nuclear Regulatory Commission as the agency responsible for licensing a facility; it directed the Environmental Protection Agency to promulgate health-based standards on which to base decisions about site suitability; and it established the Department of Energy (DOE) as the contractor responsible for finding a suitable site and building the repository. By 1985, the DOE had zeroed in on three sites: a salt site in Deaf Smith County, Texas, and two sites in volcanic rocks, one at Hanford, Washington, and one at Yucca Mountain, Nevada. While the Texas site may have been selected on its geologic merits, the Hanford and Yucca Mountain sites certainly were not. Volcanic rocks would rate far down the list of rock types most likely to provide strong containment of escaping radionuclides. The two volcanic sites were almost certainly selected on political grounds. Both are located on already established nuclear reservations where it was thought that sociopolitical opposition would be less strident.

In December 1987, the promise of full public participation went out the window. With the DOE still in the midst of a comparison of the three sites, an amendment to the Nuclear Waste Policy Act was pushed through Congress without hearings, discussions, or debate. Under this backroom deal, the programs at Deaf Smith County and Hanford were canceled. The only site that would remain under consideration as a potential nuclear repository for high-level waste would be the site at Yucca Mountain, Nevada.

The 1987 amendment was an attempt by Congress to get the nuclear waste program back on a fast track, but the fast tracking has never come to pass. The citizens of the state of Nevada were outraged, feeling that they already bear an unfair share of the nation's nuclear burden. Opinion polls in Nevada have consistently shown 75–80 percent opposition to the Yucca Mountain site.[61] The state of Nevada brought suit against the DOE, effectively closing down the project for several years. Although the program is now back in gear, it has been more than a decade since the 1987 amendment, and despite budgets in the hundreds of millions of dollars per year, the Yucca Mountain site has still not been licensed. There are now whispers heard in dark corridors that perhaps it never will be.

The source of all this fear and trepidation is the undoubted fact that radioactive emissions cause cancer in living tissue. They are carcinogenic, mutagenic, and teratogenic. As with organic chemicals, there is no doubt about the direct impact of acute exposures to certain isotopes of certain radioactive elements, but there *is* doubt about the indirect impact of long-term chronic doses at very low levels. The latter uncertainty is critical, because as we shall see, the levels of radioactivity likely to reach potential receptors from a subsurface waste repository will be very low indeed.

The concepts of exposure, dose, and dose-response are the same for radioactive contaminants as they are for organic contaminants, as described earlier, but the jargon and the units of measurement are entirely different. Total radioactivity consists of two types of subatomic particle emissions (alpha particles and beta particles) and two types of electromagnetic radiation (gamma rays and x-rays). Total radioactivity is measured in curies (given the symbol Ci), where one curie is the amount of radioactivity emitted by one gram of pure radium. Radioactivity at the level of microcuries (one-millionth of a curie), or even nanocuries (one-billionth of a curie), can be biologically important. Radioactivity at the level of megacuries (millions of curies) is produced in nuclear reactors.[62] Radionuclide concentrations in water are expressed in picocuries per liter (pCi/L). A picocurie is one-trillionth (or 10^{-12}) of a curie. Maximum permissible concentrations of radionuclides in drinking water vary from a few pCi/L (for strontium-90 and cesium-137, for example) to a few hundred pCi/L (for radon-222 and iodine 129) to a few thousand pCi/ L (for plutonium-239).

Exposure is measured in a unit with the odd designation of roentgen-equivalent-man (or rem). One rem is the amount of radiation carried by a radioactive emission that deposits a specific amount of energy in one gram of living tissue. It includes a fudge factor that accounts for the greater biological efficiency of alpha radiation relative to beta or gamma radiation. It is alpha radiation that is most harmful to human tissue. Total radiation exposure is often reported in millirems (one-thousandth of a rem).

Permissible dose levels reflect the importance of the rate of exposure and thus have units of millirems per year (mrems/y). There are many types of dose limits in use. Some specify limits for the whole body; others for specific bodily organs. Some specify limits for individuals; others for the population as a whole. Some specify limits for the public at large;

others for workers in the nuclear industry. Most of these permissible dose levels lie in the range of a few millirems to a few tens of millirems per year. The standard for strontium-90, for example, which is one of the strictest, is 4 mrems/y. The maximum permissible total dose recommended for the general public by the International Commission on Radiological Protection is 500 mrems/y.[63] At Yucca Mountain, the Energy Policy Act of 1992 directed the EPA to promulgate a site-specific radiation protection standard for the site, but as of early 1998 this regulatory guidance was still not available. The DOE has imposed an interim performance standard on itself while awaiting the EPA's decision. The department hopes to show that the repository will not deliver a dose rate greater than 25 mrems/y to potential receptors.[64]

The radioactive standards that must be met by potential environmental releases from a nuclear repository are extremely conservative. The interim Yucca Mountain performance standard of 25 mrems/y is actually smaller than the dose rate of about 100 mrems/y experienced by all of us every day from background radiation. The exposure that arises from a single chest x-ray leads to much higher dose rates than the environmental standards.

Radioactive elements differ strongly in the dose they deliver to human tissue at a given level of radioactive emissions. For each radioisotope, there is a so-called dose conversion factor, in units of rems per curie, that provides an indication of the degree of biological damage that can be expected. These dose conversion factors cover many orders of magnitude for the various radionuclides likely to emerge from a subsurface repository. It is this variation that leads to the wide spread in the maximum permissible concentrations and dose rates quoted above.

As if all this weren't complicated enough, there is a new system of units in use in most other countries. It has arisen as a part of the move toward Systeme Internationale (SI) metric units on the part of the international scientific community. In this system, the becquerrel (Bq) replaces the curie as the basic unit of radioactivity, and the sievert (Sv) replaces the rem as the unit for dose. A concentration of a radionuclide in water of 100 pCi/L converts to 3.7 Bq/L, and a dose rate of 100 rems/ y converts to 1 Sv/y. Having defined this confusing array of oddly named units in textbook fashion, let us leave them to the nuclear scientists and move on.

As we learned in an earlier chapter, a subsurface repository is a complex engineering undertaking. It involves the construction of underground shafts, drifts, adits, and rooms. The design concept is one of multiple barriers, including a strong and corrosion-resistant canister to house the spent fuel rods, low-permeability clay buffer material around the canister, and backfilling, grouting, and sealing of the underground openings. There has been much controversy about the appropriate design life to strive for, in the engineered components of a nuclear repository. Some of the radionuclides remain hazardous for millions of years, but this is an uncomfortably long period for the design engineers. No engineering facility could be guaranteed to function for millions of years. The usual engineering design framework is on the order of hundreds of years, but this is an uncomfortably short period for those who are most concerned about the health risk from escaping radionuclides. The compromise, which is now encoded in many of the regulations is 10,000 years.

Now, this is a political rather than a technical compromise, because it is not possible for engineers to design a multiple-barrier system that will last 10,000 years. It should be possible to design a system to last 100 years, and maybe 1,000, but not 10,000. So, like landfills, nuclear repositories are subject to the longevity catch. The engineered components will undoubtedly fail and release contaminants into the subsurface environment at some point in the future. The multiple-barrier system will delay the releases but it will not prevent them.

Under these circumstances, the ultimate "barrier" is the host rock in which the repository sits. Radionuclides released from the repository at Yucca Mountain will migrate through the unsaturated zone to the water table, dissolve in the ambient groundwater, and be carried by the flowing groundwater from the repository toward the accessible biosphere. Luckily, like organic contaminants, the migration of most radionuclides is highly retarded by sorption onto clay particles, organic matter, and certain minerals that tend to coat the fracture surfaces in fractured rocks at sites like Yucca Mountain. The rate of advance of the contaminants is likely to be only a fraction of the rate of flow of the groundwater. In the laboratory it has been shown that the rate of migration of strontium-90 is retarded 20-fold relative to flowing groundwater. For plutonium-239 the retardation may be as large as 2,000-fold.[65] Unfortunately, it has not yet been confirmed that these values are applicable in the field, but there seems little doubt that retardation is an important attenuating process.

The ideal site for a nuclear repository is in a rock type of very low permeability with a strong sorption potential. It should have a long travel path from the repository to the discharge point of the groundwater flow system where the radionuclides might become available to potential receptors. The WIPP site, more than 2,000 feet deep in the bedded salts of New Mexico, satisfies these criteria as well as could be expected from any site. The site at Yucca Mountain, Nevada, is not as good a site as the WIPP site. The water table at Yucca Mountain is very deep and the proposed repository horizon is above the water table in the unsaturated zone (often called the vadose zone in this project). Some people think this is a good thing; others think it is a bad thing; but there is no doubt that it adds complexity and uncertainty to the prediction of the exposure pathways. It is likely that the heat generated by the decaying radionuclides will boil the water in the host rock, driving it away in vapor form to condense elsewhere in the repository system. Current performance assessments assume that any contaminated leachates released when the canisters fail in some future century will ultimately migrate down to the water table. Groundwater travel times from the site to downstream discharge areas are on the order of thousands of years.[66] Contaminant travel times from the site to potential receptors ought to be much longer, under the retardation introduced by radionuclide sorption. The question on the table is whether the travel times will be sufficiently long to allow the radionuclides to decay to concentration levels that will meet the applicable health standards over the 10,000-year design horizon, or better yet, over a 100,000-year assessment period, which is the time frame desired by opponents of the site.

There are more than a hundred different radionuclides released from a spent fuel rod. The rate of decay of any one of them is indicated by its *half-life*. This parameter defines the length of time it takes for one gram of the radionuclide to lose half its mass through spontaneous radioactive disintegration. The range of half-lives for the different radionuclides is immense. Some fission products like strontium-90 and cesium-137 have half-lives of less than 30 years, and they decay to innocuous levels in a few hundred years. Some of the transuranic elements (elements with atomic numbers higher than uranium) such as neptunium, plutonium, and americium, have much longer half-lives. Plutonium-239, for example, has a half-life of 24,400 years. Two of the most long-lived isotopes are technicium-99, with a half-life of 210,000 years, and iodine-129, with a half-life of 16 million years. These latter radioisotopes are hazardous over periods that are orders of magnitude longer than the history of humankind.[67] If there is going to be health risk from repository leakage, it is going to arise from these very long-lived radionuclide species.

And so we approach the bottom line. The site characterization program at Yucca Mountain has been going, off and on, for more than a decade now. The DOE has brought in some of the most reputable scientific agencies in the land to carry out the work, among them the United States Geological Survey, out of their Denver office; Sandia National Laboratories, which is based in Albuquerque, New Mexico; and the National Laboratories at Los Alamos, New Mexico; Berkeley, California; and Livermore, California. These teams have studied the stratigraphy and structure of the volcanic rocks at the site; they have measured the permeability of the various hydrogeologic units; they have investigated the sorption properties of the different radionuclides; they have run field tracer tests to emulate the possible future migration of radionuclides through the hydrologic system; and they have driven a large-diameter tunnel into the repository horizon to examine things firsthand. All the data from these programs has gone into a huge database, and this database has been used to drive computer models that can predict future repository performance.

The data are far from perfect. There are uncertainties to be sure. But when all is said and done, despite the doubts about a vadose-zone site in volcanic rocks, these models predict worst-case peak dose rates for critical radionuclides that are well below the applicable radiological standards. In fact, base-case performance-assessment calculations predict that *no* dose will be experienced by potential human receptors within the 10,000-year design period. Even after the 10,000-year period, the *total* dose rate that will be experienced by any plausible receptor scenario is unlikely to exceed a few millirems per year, or a few tens of millirems per year at most.[68] Most scientific experts are convinced that the Yucca Mountain facility poses little risk to public health.[69]

Similar findings have come from other repository programs. At the WIPP site, a National Academy of Sciences committee concluded that "human exposure to radiation from the WIPP site will not exceed U.S. or international radiation protection standards."[70] A case study (but not a worst case study) carried out by Atomic Energy of Canada Limited for a potential repository in the granites of the Canadian Shield concluded that the *mean* dose rate to an individual in the critically exposed population would be six orders of magnitude less than the applicable Canadian radiological risk criteria and eight orders of magnitude less than the dose rate from natural background radiation. It is claimed that the risk will be no greater than that emanating from a naturally occurring uranium ore deposit.[71] A risk analysis carried out by the EPA for a generic repository suggests an upper bound of one death per decade attributable to exposure to repository radiation. These calculations do not identify the construction and operation of a nuclear waste repository as a particularly risky venture. H. W. Lewis, in his book *Technological Risk,* describes the nuclear waste issue as "an egregious example of an overblown risk that has paralyzed our government for years." He claims that "it is a phony issue, and it would be in the national interest to get on to more important matters."[72]

Despite all this, there is a widespread consensus across the land that perhaps the technocrats are just a wee bit too cocky.[73] All of these reassuring calculations of dose rate carry a rider stating that the calculations do not include the possibility of human intrusion into a still-percolating repository, either unintentionally, as a part of some future petroleum or mineral exploration, or purposefully, as an act of war or terrorist sabotage. In any case, the public is not all that willing to separate the waste-disposal step of the nuclear fuel cycle from the other steps, including in particular, the construction and operation of the reactors themselves. The fear is not so much of long-term chronic emissions as it is of sudden disastrous failures like Chernobyl. What should be clear from this discussion is that underground nuclear waste repositories are much less prone to disastrous failure than reactors. (Studies have shown that even earthquakes are unlikely to do much damage to subsurface workings or lead to larger releases.) It is the production end of the nuclear fuel cycle that hosts the dangers, not the waste end. If you want to oppose nuclear power and be rational about it, the issue is reactor safety, not repository safety. And it must be remembered that even if nuclear power were to suffer a complete fall from grace in the coming years (an event that seems unlikely despite recent downturns), there would still be large amounts of historical high-level waste that require "permanent" disposal. If properly sited, and this is done with care, there is no real impediment to the safe disposal of this waste.

THE BOTTOM LINE

- The widespread environmental contamination from past mismanagement of industrial waste did not occur under malicious intent. Rather, the cause of the failure was indifference, ignorance, and a lack of communication across the disciplines.

- Environmental policy should emphasize prevention of future contamination at the expense of the remediation of historical contamination. Prevention is at least an order of magnitude more cost-effective than remediation. Current EPA programs designed to prevent contamination of drinking-water aquifers, such as the Wellhead Protection Program and the Sole Source Aquifer Program, should be expanded.

- In the United States, the main preventive instrument is the RCRA legislation. While far from perfect, it has led to significant improvements in industrial practices. The weakest provisions of RCRA are the ones that limit operator liability to a period that ends 30 years after site closure. Monitoring of waste-management facilities should be required in perpetuity.

- Recycling is an important and valuable component in the mix of waste-management strategies needed to keep our waste problems under control. There is still considerable scope for the enhancement of both municipal and industrial recycling activities. However, it is not a panacea. Even under the most optimistic scenarios, recycling can handle only a small percentage of the total waste generated. It will not negate the need for the siting of new landfills for both municipal and industrial waste.

- Modern landfills, with their improved design specifications, are much less likely to leak than poorly designed older landfills, over the short term. However, even the most well-constructed landfills have a finite life expectancy, probably on the order of 50 to 100 years. Landfills delay, attenuate, and possibly reduce groundwater contamination, but they do not prevent it forever.

- The dominant process leading to the migration of contaminants from source areas into the surrounding environment involves the formation of dissolved contaminant plumes that are carried forward by flowing groundwater. The siting of waste-management facilities on low-permeability deposits would reduce the rates of plume advance so significantly that it is unlikely that contamination from such sites would ever threaten water-supply aquifers. Environmental policies that encourage proper technical siting of waste-management facilities represent the single most important step that could be taken to protect the environment from contamination.

- Unfortunately, the promise afforded by good technical siting is negated by the sociopolitical difficulties engendered by the NIMBY syndrome. None of the approaches that have been tried to achieve siting consensus have been very successful. The inability of our current political framework to successfully site needed waste-management facilities encourages unacceptable practices that expose the public to greater health risks than would accrue from properly sited facilities.

- Nuclear waste repositories also suffer from the longevity catch. The multiple-barrier designs under consideration will delay but not prevent releases to the environment. However, the radionuclides that will ultimately be released from such facilities undergo radioactive degradation and are strongly sorbed onto geological materials. While uncertainties remain, it appears that dose rates from carefully sited facilities will meet radiological standards with a large margin of safety. If done with care, there is no real impediment to the safe disposal of high-level nuclear waste. Safety issues associated with the operation of the nuclear reactors themselves are of much greater concern than those associated with subsurface nuclear waste repositories.

5 The Unpleasant Truths about Remediation

There is no question what the members of the public want at contaminated sites. They want them "cleaned up." They want them returned to the pristine conditions that existed before they were fouled by evil polluters. They want every last drop of contaminant sucked back out of the ground. They want their groundwater cleansed of all contamination and protected from the threat of all future contamination.

THE HOLY GRAIL: SITE RESTORATION THROUGH CONTAMINANT REMOVAL

Legislators at both the state and federal level have heard the message loud and clear. Almost all the early legislation, including the Superfund legislation, assumed that the goal of remedial activities was complete cleanup, or at least cleanup to a level that met all applicable health standards. It was assumed that these standards would be met at every contaminated site targeted for cleanup, and at each site they would be met both in the source area and throughout the plume. The problem was viewed as having two parts: remove the source areas, and shrink the plumes. Early programmatic goals did not question whether this could be done: they simply specified how many sites would be cleaned up under the anticipated budgets, and on what schedule.

It is hard to find fault with this way of thinking. It is in the tradition of American "can do" optimism. There is only one problem: the optimism was misplaced. It has not proven possible to clean up source areas, certainly not to pristine conditions, and in most cases, not even to the point of compliance with established health standards. The early goals were laudable, but they have turned out to be neither economically nor technically feasible.

The agents of fate in this case are the dreaded DNAPLs introduced in the last chapter. These are the free-product liquid contaminants— solvents, wood-preserving chemicals, PCB-laced oils, and pesticides— which are denser than water, and which residualize themselves below the water table in pools, blobs, and droplets within the pores and fractures of the subsurface soils and rocks. The great majority of contaminated sites in North America, and especially those of industrial origin, have residualized DNAPLs in their source area. It is our inability to remove all of the DNAPL from the subsurface, or for that matter to even locate where it all is, that has rendered most contaminated sites impossible to clean up. There are simply no current technologies that will remove every last droplet from the subsurface soils and rocks. Unfortunately, as we shall see shortly, if the source areas threaten drinking-water aquifers, then it *is necessary* to remove almost every last droplet to prevent the formation of contaminant plumes that will snake their way through these aquifers at concentrations that exceed the health standards.

My colleague John Cherry has referred to DNAPL sites as having "terminal cancer." Carrying the analogy further, he identifies the source area as the locus of the disease, the "tumor," if you will, and the plume that emanates from the source area as the "symptom." As we shall see, scientists have learned how to treat the symptoms, but as yet they have no cure for the disease.[1]

In order to get a feeling for the types of remedial measures that come under consideration at contaminated sites, we will turn to a case history.[2] Price's Landfill, near Atlantic City, New Jersey, bears many similarities to the Ville Mercier case history introduced in chapter 1. Like the one at Ville Mercier, the landfill was developed in an old sand-and-gravel quarry, and it operated in the period 1969 to 1976, before the inappropriateness of such sites was widely recognized. It accepted both solid municipal waste and liquid chemical waste, and as at Ville Mercier, there is anecdotal evidence of tanker trucks opening their spigots directly into the quarry. Price's Landfill sits over the Cohansey aquifer, about one mile west of a well field that is the primary source of water supply for the Atlantic City Municipal Water Authority. It was recognized in the late seventies that the aquifer was being contaminated by the landfill. At least one of the city pumping wells was closed down as early as 1981 under threat of contamination.

Table 15 lists some of the remedial alternatives that came under consideration at Price's Landfill[3] (together with a few that didn't). In general, the approaches fall into one of three categories: accept the risk, contain the contamination, or try to remove it.

If we decide to accept the risk, what is usually meant is that the risk is so small that we choose to do nothing about it. As we have seen in the last chapter, there are some waste-management facilities that have been fortuitously constructed in favorable hydrogeological settings, which may indeed offer very little risk to potable water supplies. In such circumstances, it may be societally optimal to accept the do-nothing option.

The risk at Price's Landfill was not small enough to consider a do-nothing option. However, we might still accept the risk in a sense if we were to decide to accept the contaminated conditions in the aquifer without attempting any remedial program in the aquifer or at the landfill. Now, it is not likely that anyone would accept the contaminated groundwater as an untreated source of supply, so there are two further options that fall under this category. We could treat the water at the

Table 15 Remedial options at Price's Landfill, Atlantic City, New Jersey.

Approach		Technology	Estimated Cost[a]
Accept the risk		Do nothing	not considered
		Wellhead treatment	not considered
		Develop alternate sources of supply	$8.5–11.3 million
Contaminant containment	Surface control	Grading and surface water control	$0.5 million
		Capping	$0.6–1.3 million
	Physical barriers and cutoff walls	Bentonite slurry trench	$1.8 million
		Grout curtain	$3.8 million
		Sheet piling	$2.2 million
	Plume management	Pump-and-treat	$4.8 million[b]
Contaminant mass removal		Pump-and-treat	$4.8 million[b]
		Excavation	$12.7 million
		Emerging technologies	not considered

[a]For the 22-acre landfill; capital costs, in 1980 dollars.
[b]Including net present value of operational costs for pumping and treatment for 20 years of operation.
Source of data used in table: Mark Sharefkin, Mordechai Schecter, and Allen Kneese, "Impacts, Costs, and Techniques for Mitigation of Contaminated Groundwater: A Review," *Water Resources Research* 20 (1984): 1771–83.

wellhead (which was not considered at Price's Landfill), or we could try to develop an alternative source of supply (which for Price's Landfill was costed out at $8.5 to $11.3 million in 1980 dollars).

For those sites where contaminant plumes have entered drinking-water aquifers, and where wellhead treatment or the development of alternate sources of supply are not acceptable options, one is left with two possibilities: try to contain the source and control the plume, or try to remove the source. In Table 15 the containment options are divided into those involving surface control, those employing physical barriers and cutoff walls, and those based on plume management. Surface control measures such as grading and capping are carried out at most contaminated sites as part of the remedial package, but not usually as the primary thrust. At many sites, physical barriers have been constructed around source areas. The technology now exists to install such barriers to depths of tens of feet (or even hundreds of feet in favorable geologic materials).

By far the most common remedial action has involved the installation of pump-and-treat systems wherein contaminated water is pumped from afflicted aquifers, treated to remove the contaminants, and then either used as a water supply, reinjected back into the aquifer, or released into lakes or streams. Note in Table 15 that pump-and-treat is listed twice, once as a plume management technology under the containment approach and once as a mass removal technology. As we shall soon see, pumping water from plume areas can be effective in controlling plume migration, whereas pumping from source areas is seldom effective in removing contaminant mass.

The only contaminant removal technology that has ever really proven itself is excavation. What could be simpler, after all, than digging up the source areas and removing the "tumors." NIMBY groups usually demand it, and regulatory agencies looking for simple solutions that will solve problems once and for all, often embrace it. For very small volumes of contaminated material, like those associated with leaking underground storage tanks, the excavation option makes good sense, but for larger contaminated sites of the Superfund variety, excavation is simply too expensive. Note in Table 15, for Price's Landfill, which at twenty-two acres is actually a very small landfill, that excavation is by far the most expensive option at $12.7 million. (And remember, these are 1980 dollars; current costs would be double or more.) At Ville Mercier, which is a bigger site, cost estimates for the excavation option ran greater than $100 million. When one begins to see cost estimates of this size, while remembering the tens of thousands of sites that exist around the country, it is reasonable to question whether the societal risk reductions achieved can possibly be worth the expense.

There is another issue associated with excavation: what to do with the excavated material. Most remedial plans specify that the excavated material should be taken to a "secure landfill." However, as we have seen, even the most secure landfill is secure only in the short term. One can easily conjure up visions of waste excavated from one site and placed in another, only to require reexcavation and reemplacement once again a few tens of years down the road. It sounds like a wonderful plan for the waste-excavation companies, but I doubt that it is optimal for society at large.

Lastly, there is the question of whether excavation necessarily reduces health risk. At Ville Mercier, for example, risk analyses indicated that the additional health risks that would be borne by local residents and on-site workers during the excavation process would be greater than those associated with just leaving the contamination in place. The activities associated with digging up toxic waste, transporting it across the countryside, and reemplacing it somewhere else are not risk-free.

The last line in Table 15 notes that none of the *emerging technologies* for contaminant mass removal were considered at Price's Landfill. Of course, the decisions at Price's Landfill were made back in the early 1980s, and there really wasn't that much emerging at the time. Surely, as we have reached the millennium, some new technologies must be coming on the scene that offer promise for contaminant removal from the subsurface. The answer is that such technologies *are* on the horizon (and some are even on the market), but the promise is still distant, not immediate. We will look at them somewhat more closely a few sections hence.

LOSS OF INNOCENCE:
THE SAD TALE OF PUMP-AND-TREAT

In the naive glow of the "can do" period following the passage of the Superfund legislation in the early 1980s, hundreds of pump-and-treat systems were put in place at contaminated sites across the nation. The idea was simple: put some wells in the ground; pump out all the contaminated liquids; treat them to remove the contaminants; and walk away. The engineering work plans for these early projects are full of optimistic calculations of the amount of time required to attain the desired cleanup standards. Most consultants and contractors promised their clients that they would be off the hook within a few months, or at most a few years.

It was not to be. The reality has been a sad tale of failure and frustration. Pump-and-treat has been so ineffective in removing contaminants from the subsurface that the results are almost laughable. At Ville Mercier for example, three wells have been pumping since 1984 at a combined rate of 700 gallons per minute. In the first eight and a half years of operation these wells pumped almost 3 billion gallons of water out of the ground. This contaminated water was then sent through a treatment plant at a cost of about $1 million per year. And what was accomplished? The total amount of all chemicals removed from the subsurface has been about 13,000 gallons, less than 0.001 percent of the water pumped. More important, the estimated volume of chemicals in the ground at Ville Mercier runs to about 4.5 million gallons, which means that the amount of chemical removed in eight and a half years of pumping is less than 1 percent of that still remaining in the ground. The cost of removal has been $650 per gallon, which is probably about one thousand times more than the chemicals were worth in the first place.

Results from across North America tell the same story. Pumping wells on the Kodak property in Rochester, New York, pump more than 5 million gallons of water per year in order to retrieve less than 1,000 gallons of TCE and methylene chloride. At the Fairchild semiconductor site in California, pumping more than a billion gallons of water per year recovers less than 2,000 gallons per year of acetone and xylene.[4]

As you have probably suspected by now, the villains in this piece are the LNAPLs and DNAPLs floating around in the groundwater beneath the sites. Pumping wells designed to pump water are simply not effective in capturing NAPLs. Some of the pumping wells in the early pump-and-treat systems were actually designed to recover NAPL pools directly. In the early years there were many articles in the technical literature suggesting various strategies to optimize direct NAPL recovery. Time and experience have taught us that even this seemingly straightforward objective is not viable. The NAPLs tend to be distributed irregularly throughout the source area in small pockets and globules not easily isolated or recovered. When the pumps are turned on, the ground-water comes into the well preferentially relative to the free-product chemicals. The residualized NAPLs resist dislodging from the nooks and crannies where they have settled; the sorbed NAPLs remain glommed onto the organic matter that now acts as their host. The water pumped out, whether it be from a plume area or a source area, contains dissolved contaminants, but because the solubilities of most of these chemicals are very low, the mass of chemical removed is just a minuscule percentage of the water pumped. Even when the contaminant concentrations are very low (measuring just a few parts per billion), they may exceed the very conservative health standards that have been set, and all the pumped water must therefore be sent through the very expensive treat-ment facilities.

In 1990, the EPA carried out a review of a large number of the pump-and-treat facilities operating under the Superfund legislation.[5] The agency's findings were uniform across the nation. Contaminant concen-trations in affected aquifers are sometimes reduced by pump-and-treat activities, but the rate of reduction tapers off as pumping proceeds; and if the pumps are stopped, concentrations usually return to their original levels. All cases show massive volumes of water pumped for minuscule contaminant recoveries. The time estimates for "cleanup" were univer-sally optimistic. In fact, it is now recognized that at most of these sites cleanup goals will never be achieved through pump-and-treat alone.

It is not only the pumping end of the pump-and-treat game that is problematical. So too is the treatment end. It will not be within the scope of this book to go into treatment issues in detail, but it is certainly worth noting here that the removal of organic chemicals from water is not a simple or straightforward task. If the contamination is limited to a single chemical, chances for success are better. Some chemicals, being volatile, are easily removed through air stripping. Others that are strongly sorbed to organic matter can be removed from the water through carbon ab-sorption technologies. In most cases, however, contamination does not consist of a single chemical. Most source areas contain a cocktail of chem-icals, all with different physical and chemical properties. It is difficult and expensive to design treatment plants that can strip out all these contaminants together. At Ville Mercier, for example, where the cocktail was particularly exotic, the $1-million-per-year treatment plant was actually quite inefficient, and the "treated" water that came out the end of the system was really only partially treated. Concentrations of many of the chemicals still exceeded health standards. Nevertheless, with regulatory approval, this water was released into a nearby surface stream. It is likely (although by no means sure) that the natural groundwater flow would have delivered the contaminated groundwater to this same stream eventually, but there is no question that it got there faster through the hand of man than it would have through the hand of nature.

Surprisingly, there is a silver lining to the pump-and-treat story. The news is not all bad. We alluded above to the role that pump-and-treat can play in the containment of groundwater contamination. Containment is a much less lofty goal than restoration, but it has the advantage that it may be attainable. Under a containment strategy no attempt is made to clean up the source zone. Instead emphasis is placed on preventing the formation of plumes that threaten to migrate into water supply aquifers. The use of physical barriers and cutoff walls to accomplish this goal was listed in Table 15. In that case the idea is simple: build a barrier around the source area and cut off access to the groundwater flow. The role of pump-and-treat in the prevention of plume migration may be less obvious. The method is based on the concept of a capture zone. Every well captures the groundwater flow from a certain volume of the aquifer it taps. If a set of wells can be installed downstream from a source area such that their capture zones encompass the source area and all potential plumes emanating from it, then the potential contaminant migration is brought under control. The control in the case of cutoff walls is physical; in the case of pump-and-treat it is hydraulic.

Many of the pump-and-treat systems put in place to try to remove contaminant mass back in the eighties have turned out to be effective as agents of plume containment in the nineties. As the paradigm has shifted from source restoration to plume management, pump-and-treat technology has come back to the forefront, except that now these systems are designed to optimize containment rather than contaminant removal.

There is one other difference between these two paradigms, and it is an important one. When viewed as a site restoration tool, pump-and-treat always had a finite time horizon, express or implied, after which it was assumed that goals would be reached and the pumps turned off. In the containment option, pump-and-treat must be viewed as perpetual. Because the source will remain forever, so too must the pumping. It remains to be seen whether governments, corporations, regulatory agencies, and the public have the will to fund and administer environmental programs that have no end.

There is another perspective on this latter issue that is perhaps not quite so pessimistic.[6] This view holds that the goal of current remediation efforts should continue to be short-term risk reduction through containment, but with the aim to pass on to future generations site conditions that are well-suited to the future application of emerging technologies with improved mass-removal capabilities, if and when such technologies arrive on the shelf.

The question is: Are such technologies on the way? Or is this just a futile hope, akin to our wish for universal peace and happiness? I will address this question shortly, but first I must ask a different question. I said earlier that source-area restoration is of little value unless we can remove almost every last drop of DNAPL. This seems like a pretty tall order. Why do we have to set such a difficult goal?

THE 99.9 PERCENT SOLUTION:
SOLUBILITY AND STANDARDS

I have continually made the point that the solubility of organic chemicals in water is very low, but that the regulatory drinking-water standards, established on the basis of avoiding a 1 in 1 million incremental increase in health risk, are lower yet. Table 16 compares these two values for a few representative organic contaminants. The regulatory standards are taken from Table 5, but the units have been converted from micrograms per liter to milligrams per liter to bring them into sync with the usual units of measurement for solubility.

(For the benefit of the metrically challenged, milligrams are 1,000

Table 16 Solubilities and regulatory standards for some
representative organic chemicals.

Contaminant	Solubility (mg/L)	Regulatory Standard (mg/L)	Multiplier
TCE	1100	0.005	220,000
Pentachlorophenol	14	0.001	14,000
PCB	31	0.0005	62,000
EDB	4300	0.00005	86,000,000
Benzene	1750	0.005	350,000

times larger than micrograms, both being very small, and a liter is about the same size as a fifth of whiskey. The highest solubility among chemicals listed in the table, for the pesticide EDB, is 4,300 mg/L. A liter of water weighs 1,000 grams, or 1,000,000 milligrams, so that a saturated solution is only 0.43 percent EDB and 99.57 percent water, hence the designation of the solubility as "low." As an example of a high solubility, consider the inorganic compound ammonia. With a solubility of 530,000 mg/L, a saturated solution is more than 50 percent ammonia.)

The difference between the solubility (which identifies the highest concentration that can be achieved in a contaminated aquifer) and the regulatory standard (which identifies the highest acceptable concentration) is indicated by the multiplier in the right-hand column of Table 16. For EDB, for example, the regulatory standard is 86 million times smaller than the solubility. In other words, if groundwater were contaminated with dissolved EDB to its solubility limit, a remedial technology would have to reduce that concentration by a factor of 86 million to bring it into compliance with the standard. For the wood-preserving chemical pentachlorophenol, which has one of the lowest multipliers of all the organic chemicals, one would still have to reduce concentrations by a factor of 14,000 to reach compliance.

It should be clear that this is a tall order. Any remedial technology designed to reduce dissolved contaminant concentrations in a groundwater plume would have to be incredibly effective to meet these concentration-reducing objectives. Of course, in a dissolved plume, if we accept containment as a suitable objective, then we could choose to rely on a pump-and-treat system designed to capture the plume before it moves too far away from the source area. In that case, concentration reduction is not an issue, because all the contaminated water, at whatever concentration, is sucked into the wells as it flows by. (That is, concentration reduction is not an issue *in the aquifer*; as we have seen, it may still be an issue *in the treatment plant*.)

It is in the source area of a DNAPL site that the huge multiplier between solubilities and standards really comes to the fore. Because of it, even a small blob of free-product chemical has the potential to dissolve into the groundwater and create concentrations that are orders of magnitude greater than the established standards. This fact has led those who have studied the problem to conclude that contaminant removal technologies need to achieve almost complete removal of all DNAPL pools, blobs, ganglia, and droplets in the source area of a contaminated site before one can begin to hope that it will no longer give birth to contaminant plumes that can bleed into surrounding aquifers.[7] If one needs a numerical value for the necessary recovery rates, the value usually quoted is 99.9 percent.

We might well ask whether such recovery rates are even remotely possible with any of the emerging technologies likely to come into play. As a starting point for such a discussion, let us look to the petroleum industry for precedents. Oil companies are trying to do the same thing in their oil fields that environmental engineers are trying to do at DNAPL-contaminated sites. They are both trying to extract as much of their target fluid as the subsurface soils and rocks are willing to give up. In the oil patch, the target fluids are oil and gas; in the environmental cleanup world, the target fluids are the solvents and pesticides that infest contaminated sites. In the oil patch, recovery rates of 40 percent are considered cause for celebration. The industry has been experimenting for years with techniques of secondary recovery that are designed to improve performance. In fact, many of the emerging technologies that I will introduce in the next section had their genesis as secondary-recovery efforts in the petroleum industry. But even with these enhanced techniques, petroleum recovery rates seldom exceed 50 percent, certainly nowhere near the 99.9 percent we are seeking.

One might well argue that petroleum engineers face a more difficult challenge than environmental engineers. After all, the fluids they seek are much deeper, and they invariably occur in fractured rocks—and it is inherently more difficult to extract fluids from such rock than from the near-surface sand-and-gravel deposits that so often host environmental fluids. Still, on the basis of this argument, 99.9 percent looks like a distant goal. To see just how distant it is, we have to look more closely at how some of these emerging technologies actually work.

SCIENTISTS AND SNAKE OIL SALESMEN

I recently attended a large convention in Las Vegas dedicated to site restoration. Here one could see the two firmaments of the environmental world tiptoeing around one another in an uneasy alliance. In the upstairs lecture halls one could listen to the professors holding forth on the latest results of their laboratory research: careful studies full of chemical formulas, complex equations, and computer graphics. Small crowds of like-minded colleagues listened carefully to the encouraging aspects of the research results, but they also probed for the experimental weaknesses, the unstated assumptions, and the hidden flaws. Heated discussions accompanied many of the talks as these leaders of the research community tried to assess the real-world applicability of these laboratory dreams.

Downstairs in the massive showrooms of the Las Vegas Convention Center were the environmental entrepreneurs. Here, there were huge drill rigs for sale at half a million dollars a pop. Rows and rows of booths with names like EnviroTech and GeoMetrics and UniData displayed the instruments of environmental cleanup: filters, sensors, loggers, samplers, and pumps; hydraulic systems, thermal heaters, and huge trenching machines. Down here the crowds were thick and enthusiasm was running high. The booths featured the latest in graphic design and see-how-it-works, do-it-yourself displays. There were gimmicky advertising

Table 17 Status of emerging technologies for in situ site cleanup.

| Approach | Technology | Mechanism[a] | Phase[b] | LNAPLs | DNAPLs | | | Pesticides | Metals and Radionuclides |
				Petroleum Hydrocarbons	Chlorinated Organic Solvents	Wood-Preserving Chemicals	PCBs		
Enhanced recovery	Waterflooding	H	D	X	X	X	?	?	X
	Steamflooding	H,T	D,N	?	?	?	?	?	
	Surfactant flushing	C	D,N	?	?	?	?	?	NA
	Cosolvent flushing	C	D,N	X	?	X	?		NA
	Air sparging	C	D	X	X	?	NA		NA
In situ destruction	Thermal destruction	T	D,N	?	?	?	?	?	
	Chemical reaction	C	D,N		?	?	?		?
	Reactive barriers	C	D	NA	X	NA	NA		X
	Engineered bioremediation	B	D	X	?	?	?	?	

[a]H = Hydraulic, T = Thermal, C = Chemical, B = Biological.
[b]D = Effective for dissolved-phase contamination in plume area; N = Effective for NAPL contamination in source area.

X = Applicable technology; commercially available.
? = Technology exists in experimental status; not commercially available.
NA = Technology not applicable.
Blank = Insufficient information available.

give-aways and eye-catching, computer-generated technical charts done up in bold colors. Bold claims, too. "Zero Contamination Liners." "The Terminator for Free-Product Recovery." "Instant Containment Anywhere, Anytime." One really had to wonder whether all these folks doing deals on their napkins downstairs even knew that there was a group of folks upstairs questioning whether any of this stuff would ever work.

As outlined in Table 17, there are just two generic approaches that can possibly lead to the levels of site cleanup that might make a difference.[8] Some of the emerging technologies are designed to produce enhanced recovery of contaminants by making adaptations to the traditional pump-and-treat approach. Others are aimed at in situ destruction of the contaminants in the ground, without the need for subsequent recovery.

The five enhanced recovery technologies listed on the top half of Table 17 all involve the addition of injection wells to complement the pumping wells that form the basis of more traditional pump-and-treat systems. The injection wells are used to introduce additional fluids (water, air, steam, solvents, or surfactants) into the contaminated region in an attempt to mobilize the contaminants and remove them from the subsurface. Some of the technologies target the dissolved-phase contamination in the plume areas. Others target the NAPLs in the source areas. The goal with respect to the NAPLs is to displace them, dissolve them, or volatilize them under the hydraulic, chemical, or thermal effect of the injected fluids. It is hoped that they will be dislodged from their immobile positions as residualized or sorbed mass and carried away to the pumped wells for aboveground treatment.

Waterflooding enhances recovery through the simple expedient of injecting additional water into the system, thus increasing the hydraulic gradients and velocities of the flowing groundwater. It has a long history in secondary-recovery efforts in the petroleum industry. *Steamflooding* combines the hydraulic effects of waterflooding with the thermal effects of steam. The heat introduced into the system volatilizes some of the contaminants into the air phase and increases the amount of dissolution into the water phase. It produces a rolling condensation front that pushes the contaminated fluids toward the collection wells.[9] Surfactants are

degreasing agents. They are the magic ingredients in dish-washing de-
tergents that lift the grease from the plates in those ads on TV. They serve
the same purpose in enhanced recovery through *surfactant flushing,* pry-
ing the NAPLs out of their nooks and crannies by decreasing the inter-
facial tensions that hold them there and increasing their solubility in
water.[10] *Cosolvent flushing* is based on the fact that some organic contaminants are orders of magnitude more soluble in low-concentration solutions of certain solvents than they are in water alone.[11] *Air sparging* is
the direct injection of air into contaminated aquifers. Some volatile organic contaminants are mobilized into the air stream, which is then removed from the system with soil vapor recovery wells.[12]

The ability of these various technologies to handle specific contaminants depends on the properties of the contaminants as summarized
back in Table 14. Air sparging and steamflooding are most effective for
the more volatile contaminants. Surfactants and cosolvents work best
with the more soluble contaminants.

Perusal of the top half of Table 17 indicates that waterflooding and
air sparging are commercially available technologies, at least for some
contaminant groups. Steamflooding, surfactant flushing, and cosolvent
flushing, on the other hand, are still at the experimental stage of development. There are some encouraging laboratory results in hand for these
technologies, and field pilot-tests are under way. For example, a steamflooding pilot test carried out at the Lawrence Livermore National Laboratory in Livermore, California, successfully recovered 7,600 gallons of
gasoline from a surficial sand-and-gravel aquifer at the site. All NAPLs
were apparently removed, and dissolved concentrations of ethylbenzene, toluene, and xylene (but not benzene) were reduced below their
MCLs.[13] A surfactant pilot test carried out at the Borden test site in Ontario removed the majority of the solvent perchloroethylene (PCE) from
the test cell but left significant contaminant concentrations (including
some DNAPL) in some portions of the cell.[14] All of the field pilot-tests
and most of the laboratory tests have been carried out in homogeneous
high-permeability sands and gravels, which offer the best chance of success. Successful testing of enhanced-recovery technologies at sites with
complex geological conditions, or at sites involving contaminated fractured rocks, is still a distant dream.

None of these technologies come cheap. Cost estimates made by the EPA in 1994 show all of them to run in the range of $50–$150 per cubic yard.[15] For large contaminated sites of the Superfund variety, anticipated remedial costs are likely to run between $25–$100 million per site.

More critically, none of the enhanced-recovery methodologies have ever been shown to be capable of removing contaminant mass from the subsurface at anywhere near the target level of 99.9 percent. There are a variety of reasons. The primary one relates to the heterogeneity of most soils and rocks. The fluid flushed through the system, regardless of whether it is water, air, steam, or chemicals, tends to find the most permeable pathways. While a given methodology may well remove most of the contaminants from these pathways, it is not likely to penetrate effectively into the lower-permeability soils and rocks. The contaminants that have migrated into these formations remain untouched, free to bleed back into the cleansed parts of the system once the remedial operation is closed down. Second, there is a strong potential for some of the mobilized contaminants to escape capture by the collection system and migrate into previously uncontaminated portions of the hydrogeological system. Third, in the case of surfactants and cosolvents, the technologies can be seen as removing one chemical by replacing it with another. Unless the flushing chemicals are biodegradable or easily flushed themselves, unacceptable impacts to the subsurface environment may remain. Last, there is the question of whether total cleansing can ever be achieved through flushing, even under ideal circumstances. Downstairs in the Las Vegas Convention Center the entrepreneurs made their sales pitches to potential clients by telling them how much contaminant they would be able to remove; upstairs the scientists worried about how much would be left behind.

Given the recognized limitations of enhanced recovery, the pot of gold at the end of the rainbow (at least that's what the entrepreneurs hope for) is now thought to take the form of in situ destruction. The bottom half of Table 17 indicates four technologies that have some potential for destroying contaminant mass in place. Of course, any high school science student can tell you that mass cannot truly be destroyed. What we are actually talking about here is conversion of the mass, through thermal, chemical, or biological reactions, from harmful, toxic compounds (like benzene or TCE or EDB) into innocuous, nontoxic compounds (like water and carbon dioxide).

The *thermal destruction* technology, which is listed first on the bottom half of Table 17, is a widely used, commercially available technology for the aboveground decontamination of excavated soils, but its use in situ is problematical. In the aboveground application, it involves heating soils in thermal treatment chambers to temperatures of 1,800 to 2,100 degrees Fahrenheit (which is four or five times higher than the hottest setting on your oven). The contaminants are literally cooked right out of the soils. For in situ applications, it is necessary to bring in-place contaminated soils up to these very high temperatures by means of heating elements installed on the ground surface.[16] The method is inordinately expensive for all but the smallest and shallowest cases of site contamination, and there are obvious limitations in trying to apply this technology in the midst of currently active industrial or commercial sites.

Methods that try to encourage favorable *chemical reactions* at depth involve the injection of chemicals into the ground to oxidize or reduce the offending contaminants into less toxic daughter products. Solutions of a class of chemicals known as permanganates, long used in aboveground wastewater treatment, have been used in pilot tests to treat TCE- and PCE-contaminated soils. More exotically, laboratory tests have shown that the chemical known to nutritionists as vitamin B_{12} can be used together with certain enzymes to destroy some types of organic solvents.[17] Flushing systems designed to enhance chemical reactions suffer the same limitations as those designed to enhance recoveries: they may not penetrate into low-permeability formations, and they can get away from you. While the theory is promising, the practice will be more difficult.

A clever ploy to circumvent the flushing problem has recently come into practice. It is the use of *reactive barriers* (also known as treatment walls, treatment curtains, and funnel-and-gate systems).[18] The idea is to construct a vertical, impermeable cutoff wall, similar to those used for the physical containment of source areas but with one or more permeable sections along its length. The impermeable parts of the wall funnel the flow of contaminated groundwater through the permeable openings. Chemicals are introduced into the permeable sections of the wall, and it acts as the host for the chemical reactions that destroy the contaminants as the water flows past. One of the earliest applications used nothing more than iron filings in the treatment wall to mediate the destruction of organic solvents.[19] This technology is now commercially available and has been used at several sites across the country. The method is really a combination of containment and destruction. Rather than going after the source zone, as most destruction technologies attempt to do, it prevents the downstream migration of dissolved plumes. It provides containment by chemical means rather than by physical barriers or hydraulic control.

BUGS TO THE RESCUE: THE BIOREMEDIATION OPTION

By far the most well-developed and widely applied destruction technology is *engineered bioremediation*. Who would have thought that bacteria and viruses, those tiny microorganisms that most of us equate with disease, might come to our rescue?

The concept is very simple. These little "bugs" like to eat organic chemicals. Our industrial waste is their nutrient. All that is required is that we bring the right culture of microorganisms into contact with the right contaminants under the right conditions to keep them happy. In principle, it is a self-controlling system. As long as there are organic contaminants around, the bugs should thrive and multiply; once they have eaten all the organic contaminants, the populations should die out.

The process by which microorganisms degrade organic chemicals is known as biodegradation. It is a process that has proven most effective in environments rich in oxygen. It is also more effective for some organic chemicals than others, in particular for the BTEX compounds (benzene, toluene, ethylbenzene, and xylene) that make up gasoline. For these reasons, attempts to use the biodegradation process as the basis for engineered bioremediation has its longest history in the cleanup of gasoline spills. Not only is gasoline easily degraded, but it is also an LNAPL likely to be found floating on the water table, right below the unsaturated zone with its abundant supply of oxygen in the soil air.

The idea is not new. The first reported bioremediation system was apparently installed more than twenty-five years ago to clean up a pipeline spill in Pennsylvania.[20] In recent years, spurred on by the Superfund and the many state regulations requiring the cleanup of leaking underground storage tanks, there has been a huge growth in commercial availability of the technology (hence the X under the "petroleum hydrocarbon" column in Table 17). Because the biochemical reactions that accompany the degradation of petroleum hydrocarbons are so sensitive to the presence or absence of oxygen, the commercial systems emphasize the circulation of oxygenated water through the contaminated zone. The circulation is accomplished through the use of injection-recovery systems similar to the ones used in the various flushing technologies. Unfortunately, the bioreclamation systems are subject to the same overriding limitation as the other injection systems: they tend to circulate the oxygenated water through the high-permeability pathways and do not necessarily reach contamination that has diffused into the lower-permeability soils and rocks. Nevertheless, bioremediation of petroleum spills is an attractive remedial alternative. It is likely to be less costly than the other emerging technologies; it can often reach cleanup goals more quickly than other methods; and it is not likely to lead to mobilization and escape of contaminated fluids.

Biodegradation is effective for both dissolved and sorbed contaminants in a groundwater plume. None of the other emerging technologies are likely to be as effective in removing sorbed contamination. However, it is not effective in the direct removal of free-product NAPLs. The microorganisms are delighted to feed on the low-concentration contaminants in the dissolved plume, but like humans, they find the NAPLs toxic. Engineered bioremediation must therefore be seen as a plume-migration-control technology, rather than as a technology for the restoration of source areas.

The idea that subsurface microorganisms might be munching on gasoline spills first came to the attention of researchers when the plumes from some of these spills unexpectedly stopped migrating for no apparent reason. Even the possible impacts of contaminant sorption onto organic soils could not account for the observed attenuation. Eventually, laboratory studies confirmed that the observed attenuation was due to microbial activity. In these cases, the naturally occurring microbial populations in the soil were fortuitously amenable to using the spilled contaminants as nutrients. It is now the hope of every polluter that his or her site will be one of the lucky ones where *natural attenuation* (sometimes called *intrinsic bioremediation*) will solve all the problems without the massive costs associated with site remediation.

At sites where engineered bioremediation has been used, it is because the native populations of microorganisms have not proven effective on their own. In an engineered system, specially designed microbial mixes ("designer bugs," if you will) are injected into the system along with the oxygenated water in order to instigate or improve biodegradation rates.

The real issue on the table these days is whether bioremedial technologies can be expanded to treat other organic contaminants, like solvents and PCBs and pesticides. Most of these contaminants are DNAPLs rather than LNAPLs, and as such they tend to sink deeper into the ground into nonoxygenated territory, where biodegradation is less likely to be effective. In addition, there is the question of whether suitable microbial mixes can be designed for these chlorinated organic compounds. The latest word from the research community is cautiously optimistic. Laboratory studies are encouraging, and several field pilot-tests have been reported in the scientific literature. At the Laramie Tie Plant site in Laramie, Wyoming, for example, pilot test results showed that in the most permeable soils nearest to the point of delivery of the oxygenated water, concentrations of the wood-preserving chemicals creosote and pentachlorophenol were reduced from very high initial values to values well below health standards (in fact, they were below detection in this part of the test cell).[21] However, the pilot test also illustrated the problems associated with preferential flow paths. Many small zones of low-permeability soils remained essentially untreated. Based on these mixed findings, it was projected that full-scale subsurface bioreclamation would require a flow-through rate for oxygenated water of 15 million gallons per day, and would require an operational period of at least 250 years. While the Laramie experiments confirmed the ability of subsurface bioreclamation to reduce contaminant levels, they also raised concerns regarding the technical practicability of the technology for heavy chlorinated organics.

KISSING YOUR SISTER: THE MOVE TOWARD
SITE CONTAINMENT AND AQUIFER PROTECTION

Within the EPA and the state agencies, there has been slow but grudging acceptance of the technical impracticability of source-area cleanup through contaminant mass removal. In the Superfund program a specific guidance document has been issued to this effect.[22] It specifies the very stringent set of conditions under which responsible parties may abandon their efforts at source-area restoration. Of course, permission to back off from cleanup is always coupled with strong requirements for site containment and plume management. As I have noted in this chapter, there are several viable technologies available for the containment of dissolved plumes: hydraulic control through pump-and-treat, physical control through cutoff walls around source areas, chemical control through funnel-and-gate reactive barriers, and biological control through engineered bioremediation.

While the need for a new paradigm that emphasizes containment rather than restoration has been recognized by regulatory agencies, it has not been embraced by environmental groups and the public at large. They see this shift in emphasis as a huge cop-out on the part of large, rich, high-tech corporations, whom they believe ought to be able to find ways to unfoul their nests. Ted Smith, the executive director of the Silicon Valley Toxics Coalition, founded in 1980 to monitor the electronics industry and the agencies that regulate it, sees the end of active cleanup as "a very dangerous precedent." He is quoted in the *San Francisco Examiner* in 1996: "We know it's very sophisticated. And we know it takes time. But the companies should find technologies that can clean up their mess. They shouldn't be trying to walk away from their responsibilities."[23]

I recently saw an editorial-page cartoon in a Southern California newspaper that captures the spirit of the public mood.[24] It featured three panels, labeled "Yesterday," "Today," and "Tomorrow." "Yesterday" shows a bunch of leaky drums sitting in a black, gooey mess on the ground. "Today" has a group of men in suits carrying briefcases and wearing hard hats pointing at the mess and making notes on clipboards. "Tomorrow" shows the mess still there, but with a rickety wire fence around it and a sign that reads "Pollution Containment Zone." In the background one can see the men in suits gleefully running off into the distance.

While these public concerns run against the grain of technical and economic reality, they are certainly not irrational. We have noted earlier that in cases where the source is not removed, plume management has to be viewed as a perpetual commitment. It is not clear whether corporations, or for that matter regulatory agencies, have really bitten this bullet. The public may not understand all the nuances, but it is left with an uneasy feeling that the people in charge do not yet have their hands fully around the problem.

The current status of site restoration technologies raises a philosophical issue that often emerges during negotiations between regulators and the parties responsible for site remediation. Regulators often argue that any amount of contaminant removal, even if well short of the target value of 99.9 percent, is beneficial because it moves the site closer to restoration and therefore provides some inherent future benefit. The responsible parties argue that partial contaminant removal is no better than none in terms of the reduction of human-health risk over the foreseeable future. As John Cherry and his coauthors note, "The degree to which today's society should allocate financial resources to mass removal efforts to achieve undefinable benefits for future society is the essence of a debate that is tied to both financial and ethical issues."[25]

THE BOTTOM LINE

- In order to be effective in preventing the migration of contaminant plumes into drinking-water aquifers, cleanup technologies that attempt to remove contaminants from DNAPL source areas would have to achieve recovery rates near 99.9 percent. There are no current or emerging technologies that meet this target. Source area restoration is neither technically nor economically feasible, nor is it likely to become so in the foreseeable future.

- There are some contaminated sites that are fortuitously located in favorable hydrogeological settings and that offer very little risk to drinking-water supplies. There are other sites where natural biodegradation of petroleum hydrocarbon contaminants has led to sufficient attenuation of plume migration to eliminate the threat of aquifer contamination. In either of these circumstances, it may be societally optimal to accept the limited risk associated with such sites and allow the no-action alternative.

- At those sites where these favorable circumstances are not present, remediation efforts should focus on source containment and plume management. Fortunately, this is a viable objective that can be met through application of one of several commercially available technologies. At most sites it is now possible to attain hydraulic control through the installation of pump-and-treat systems, physical control through the construction of cutoff walls, chemical control through the use of reactive barriers, or biological control through engineered bioremediation.

- Site containment without source removal requires a commitment on the part of both corporations and regulatory agencies to maintain control in perpetuity. It remains to be seen whether these organizations and the public have the will to fund and administer environmental programs that must go on forever.

6 The Regulatory Quagmire

In the best of all worlds, every government regulation, and of particular interest to us, every environmental regulation, would be comprehensive, logical, practical, politically acceptable, cost-efficient, simple to administer, and fair. In this ideal world, every regulation would lead to benefits that outweigh the costs, both for society as a whole and for every individual in it.

There are a variety of reasons why this ideal world does not reflect the real world. Unfortunately, not every regulation is based on a careful assessment of its costs and benefits. In the environmental world, the enactment of many regulations has been driven by the response of the press and the public to environmental accidents like those at Three Mile Island and Love Canal. This is not a recipe for good regulation. Former

EPA chief William Reilly has described it as regulation "by episodic panic."[1]

REGULATIONS AND THE ZERO-SUM SOCIETY

The hope that all individuals in society will benefit from a given regulation is not tenable. As the economist Lester Thurow has pointed out in his book *The Zero-Sum Society*, regulations don't create wealth, they just redistribute it. With every regulation enacted, there are winners and losers. Some individuals gain from the provisions of the legislation and some lose.[2] To quote Thurow, "On average, society may be better off, but this average hides a large number of people who are much better off and a large number of people who are much worse off. If you are among those who are worse off, the fact that someone else's income has risen by more than yours has fallen is of little comfort." Those whose income has risen (like the purveyors of site restoration services in the case of the Superfund) have a vested interest in keeping the regulations in place, and they will lobby hard to this end. Those whose incomes have fallen (like the responsible parties that must pay the site restoration costs) have a vested interest in seeing the regulations softened, and they will work just as hard to try and drive the political process in their direction. Every regulation sows the seeds of future dispute.

Most people are not used to thinking of a clean environment as an economic commodity, but one can view environmentalism as a demand for goods and services (uncontaminated aquifers, for example) that does not differ from other consumption demands, except that it can only be achieved collectively.[3] Of course, money spent on a clean environment is not available for other purchases, and the question then arises as to whether environmental regulations raise or lower our overall standard of living. The answer is a personal one. The benefits may have a high value for some groups within society (environmentalists and outdoor recreation lovers, for example) and a lower value for other groups (such as the inner-city poor, who might prefer that public monies be spent on housing or job creation instead).

Regulations are put in place to solve problems. They are often enacted in response to public distress. The major environmental legislation (Safe Drinking Water Act, RCRA, Superfund) arose in response to public perceptions that the environment was being badly degraded. The benefits of environmental regulation (clean drinking water, reduced health risk, aesthetic pleasures) are usually understood by the public, and even if they are not, one can count on the sponsoring politicians to sing their praises in every speech. What is not always as clear to the public, and is seldom mentioned by the politicians, is that regulations cost money. There are government costs, funded by tax dollars, in the development, administration, and enforcement of regulations; and there are costs that must be borne by the regulated community, which we have seen in the case of environmental restoration can be considerable. The regulated community will of course pass these latter costs onto the consumer, so all of the costs associated with regulations are ultimately borne by each individual citizen, either through taxes or consumer prices.

It has long been argued by economists that the deliberations over proposed regulations should be accompanied by a cost-benefit analysis that attempts to relate the social costs to the benefits likely to accrue. However, only in the last decade or so has this become standard government practice (at least for those regulations not rushed into service under an "episodic panic"). Both the Superfund and RCRA predate the cost-benefit era. One can't help but wonder how different they might be had cost-benefit analysis been carried out. If one thinks back to chapter 3, and in particular to the values in Table 10 for the costs per life saved for various risk-reducing regulations, it seems clear that many of the early environmental regulations would not have survived cost-benefit analysis in their current form.

Mind you, this discussion is not meant to imply that cost-benefit analysis is either easy or value-free.[4] Back in chapter 2 I discussed the difficulties in setting time horizons and discount rates to carry out economic analysis for individual environmental projects. These issues are even more problematical when one tries to make an economic analysis of a social policy. How do we set a time horizon on assessing the effectiveness of regulations? What is a reasonable social discount rate? How do we balance the costs and benefits to the current generation with those of future generations? To these questions we must add the thorny issue, also discussed back in chapter 2, of how to put an economic value on health and life. How should we credit dollars spent toward lives saved?

There are no easy answers to these questions, and in any case we are in the hands of those in power, who have been given the right to carry out the assessments. One has to assume in a democratic society that the elected representatives reflect current societal views on such issues as the need for income redistribution, the value of life, and the value of bequeathing a clean environment to future generations.

With all the above as a rather lengthy introduction, we come to the question at hand. In the context of environmental contamination, are we underregulated or overregulated? Arguments that we are underregulated come from the environmental camp. In their point of view, environmental regulation involves a balancing act between doing favors for industrial producers and protecting public consumers.[5] The producers worry that restrictive regulations will keep them from profitably marketing worthwhile consumer products whose production need not cause environmental degradation, while consumers worry that lax regulations will allow products to be marketed that are unsafe and that will in fact lead to human health impacts and environmental degradation. The environmental viewpoint argues that regulation must be designed to minimize the public risk rather than the industry risk. Environmentalists see it as more important to protect citizens from public hazards than to attempt to enhance their welfare with risky consumer goods. On these grounds they oppose nuclear power and they want to rein in the chemical industry. They demand full site restoration at contaminated sites. They deliver strong political support for maintaining or enhancing the current heavy regulatory presence in environmental protection.

Arguments that we are overregulated come thick and fast from conservative think tanks and representatives of the private sector. Philip Howard, in his book *The Death of Common Sense*, begins his discussion of this issue by noting that the EPA alone has more than ten thousand pages of regulations in place, and that the agency's benzene rules are longer than the U.S. Constitution.[6] In the new-right viewpoint, regulation is seen as a painless way for politicians to advance public policy without having to resort to taxation. Proponents of this view feel that the public is duped into accepting regulations in situations where direct taxation would provoke a public outcry. They believe that if the public knew the true cost of these regulations, many of the more expensive ones would never receive public support. In their opinion, even some of the much-needed and well-intentioned environmental legislation tends to go too far. As an example they quote a National Academy of Sciences study that assessed the effectiveness of regulations designed to control PCBs. The study found that 99.9 percent of the regulatory control comes from a very few effective regulations, but that the total cost of PCB control is then doubled by the existence of several other regulations that attempt to control the remaining 0.1 percent.[7]

So who is right?

The answer to this question depends heavily on the jurisdiction. In the United States, at the state level, environmental regulation is often too weak; at the federal level, it is often too strong. In Canada, at both the federal level and in the most populous province of Ontario, the regulatory climate is much softer than in any of the jurisdictions in the United States. But underregulated or overregulated, the argument can easily be made that we are poorly regulated. The regulations, and more important, the administration of these regulations, do not reflect the facts as we have uncovered them. Current environmental regulations place strict controls on some chemicals that are not truly a threat to health. They enforce standards that are unreasonably stringent. They force remediation at contaminated sites that do not constitute a significant risk to society. And they demand the deployment of expensive technologies that do not work. They are designed to reduce risks to a much lower level than those found acceptable in other walks of life.

This list of grievances reflects the recent historical tendency toward overregulation in matters associated with the siting of waste-disposal facilities and the remediation of contaminated sites. However, let's get a few things straight. My arguments are not meant to provide support for wholesale environmental deregulation. The current state of overregulation has an honorable heritage. It was put in place by legislators on behalf of the environmentalist viewpoint at a time when the scope of the dangers to society was much less clear than it is today. There is no shame in overresponding to new problems in order to get your arms around them, before backing off to a more equitable position. What is needed is not repeal of environmental legislation but fine-tuning. There are five specific issues: (1) the need to reevaluate the Priority Pollutants List, with an eye to removing some of the more benign toxicants from it; (2) the need to relax the maximum contaminant levels (MCLs) for many chemicals; (3) the need to replace MCL-driven cleanups at contaminated sites with risk-based decision processes; (4) the need to bring acceptable-risk levels in environmental matters into balance with the risk levels accepted in other walks of life; and (5) the need to move from source-area restoration technologies toward containment technologies that protect drinking-water aquifers from contamination.

There will always be a need for a strong regulatory presence in environmental matters. The economic drivers that corporate management must contend with will not allow them to properly address environmental problems without government control. I worry that the current thrusts toward deregulation are too ideological. This is not an ideological matter; it is a practical matter. We need regulations that provide sufficient protection to the environment, but that do not waste valuable societal resources that would be better spent in other areas. While I support (indeed, argue for) the necessary rationalizations of the regulatory process, I worry that the current thrust toward deregulation is going to swing the pendulum far past the balance point where we would like it to come to rest. We need the pendulum to swing back a bit, but we need to dampen its tempo quickly.

MISSING CONNECTIONS

In the San Fernando Valley of California, just over the Hollywood Hills from Los Angeles, a million people get their water supply from a thick alluvial aquifer of sand and gravel that fills the valley. Making this system work takes care. For several decades now the Office of the Watermaster for the Upper Los Angeles River Area has kept tabs on the hundreds of water companies and municipal water-supply authorities in the valley in order to insure that pumping rates do not exceed the natural yield of the aquifer. The watermaster works in a complex legal environment. It is necessary to keep track of the many water-trade agreements in place between the various communities in the valley, as well as a host of water adjudications that have come from past court settlements. It is a real success story. The San Fernando aquifer system has served a growing population without suffering the precipitous water-table declines that have occurred elsewhere under similar hydrogeologic and demographic circumstances.

As fate would have it, the San Fernando Valley also hosts a thriving aerospace industry located around the Burbank airport. Hundreds of large and small companies, including the giant Lockheed Aeronautical Systems, have used solvents in growing abundance since the end of World War II. These solvents have contaminated the very aquifers used for regional water supply. There are many sources and many plumes, some of them many miles long. When the Superfund legislation was passed, the San Fernando Valley was one of the first sites placed on the National Priorities List.

All of a sudden there was a new player in town. The EPA arrived on the watermaster's turf with the weight of this very powerful federal law behind it, and began issuing orders to the polluting companies to set up pump-and-treat systems to prevent the further spread of their contaminants through the aquifer. The watermaster's office was well aware of the contamination, because several of the large municipal wells under its jurisdiction had already been closed down, but the watermaster's approach when faced with a water shortage due to the closure of contaminated wells had generally been to approve the installation of new wells in uncontaminated portions of the aquifer. It was the EPA's opinion that this strategy led to unwarranted spreading of the contaminants throughout the aquifer. The agency felt that the capture zones of the new wells were likely to suck the contaminant plumes into previously uncontaminated parts of the aquifer and compromise the effectiveness of the carefully designed pump-and-treat systems.

Moreover, it argued, why not use the treated water from the pump-and-treat systems for water supply? They would be pumping it anyway and otherwise had nothing to do with it, other than pump it back into the aquifer. It would be offered to the water companies at a good price; it would negate the need for new wells; and it would protect the integrity of the pump-and-treat systems. There was only one problem. The water companies didn't think they could sell it to their users. Why would individual householders be willing to accept treated toxic wastewater when the companies' own alternative promised delivery of the same clean water they had always enjoyed?

It was a classic case of missing connections. There was no legal or administrative mechanism to bring these parties together. For many years they danced carefully around one another with almost no contact. The watermaster's sole responsibility is water supply; the EPA's sole responsibility is water quality. What was needed of course was a basin-wide water-management plan that took both issues into account. In recent years there have been some moves toward reconciliation of the two parties. It has been recognized that both camps are better served by cooperation than by conflict. The fact remains however that there is no agency with overall authority to work out and enforce an optimal water-management strategy.

San Fernando is not an isolated case. There are similar situations all across the nation. Water-supply authorities are usually long-established and mandated at the state or municipal level. When environmental degradation occurs, federal programs kick in and never the twain shall meet.

The lack of integrated environmental policies shows up in other ways. For example, most industries discharge treated effluent from their on-site wastewater-treatment plants to surface waterways under the National Pollution Discharge Elimination System (NPDES).[8] They are required to obtain an NPDES permit (or state equivalent) that prescribes what pollutants they can legally discharge into the surface waterways and how much of each of them can be discharged. The maximum allowable discharges are supposedly calculated to insure that they will not lead to environmental degradation in the surface waterways. The permits also include strict sampling and testing protocols to insure compliance with the permits.

The NPDES permit system predates the enactment of RCRA and the Superfund legislation. When the latter two came on-line, they mandated essentially zero-tolerance for the natural spring-flow of contaminated groundwater into surface waterways. In the interpretation of the statutes, the Superfund branch of the EPA has forced companies to install expensive remedial pump-and-treat systems to prevent the discharge of very small groundwater flows at very low concentrations into rivers. At the same time, the NPDES branch of the EPA is permitting much larger flows at much higher concentrations from treatment plants on the same sites. At the Kodak plant in Rochester, New York, for example, negotiations continue regarding groundwater inflows that both sides agree will deliver contaminant mass to the Genessee River that is orders of magnitude less than that already allowed under Kodak's state pollution discharge permit. One can argue about which of the two regulatory strategies is the correct one with respect to pollutant discharges into rivers, permitted releases or zero tolerance, but no matter which side of that fence you sit on, it is impossible to defend this degree of inconsistency in regulatory policy.

Another area where integrated national policies are missing is in the trade-off between water pollution and air pollution. Landfills pollute groundwater; incinerators pollute the atmosphere. Both are allowed under regulatory control. However, there is generally no integrated assessment as to which approach is appropriate in a given setting, or what mix is appropriate in different settings. In New York City, for example, there were eleven large municipal incinerators and thousands of small residential incinerators in operation in the 1950s.[9] In the 1960s, when new air emission standards came on-line, 50 percent of the municipal incinerators and 90 percent of the residential incinerators were shut down. At the same time, as we have seen earlier, the number of landfills in New York City was being drastically reduced, ultimately to just one, the massive Fresh Kills landfill on Staten Island. Under its design inadequacies, which I discussed previously, Fresh Kills delivers a huge load of contaminants into New York Harbor every day. The final result of this decades-long evolution of New York's waste-disposal practices has been to transfer contaminants from the atmosphere to the harbor. Now this may represent a good societal decision or a bad one. But the fact remains that it was never analyzed as such. It happened by piecemeal change to several different regulations administered by different agencies without real integration. Many of the consequences were unintended, and if they turn out to be for the best, it is really nothing more than good luck.

To end this section on a more positive note, there is another case of unintended consequences that is now receiving attention. The so-called brownfields syndrome refers to tracts of formerly industrialized urban land in the downtown cores of our cities that often lie dormant, stigmatized because they are marginally contaminated with chemical waste. Until recently, developers have been unwilling to expose themselves to the environmental liability inherent in trying to clean up and develop these properties. Instead companies tended to locate their new facilities in uncontaminated suburban and rural areas, thus exposing new sites to potential contamination while the old sites lay unused and abandoned.

With their brownfields initiatives, the EPA and many state agencies are attempting to reverse this trend, encouraging redevelopment by releasing developers from fear of third-party liability.[10] Where voluntary cleanup is carried out in good faith, some agencies are now willing to sign covenants with developers and purchasers removing legal liability for past contamination. In addition, they are approving cleanup levels that are reasonable for future industrial use of the properties, rather than trying to return them to pristine conditions. In Rhode Island, brownfields initiatives have been a cooperative venture between the Rhode Island Department of Environmental Management and the Rhode Island Economic Development Corporation,[11] thus providing the environmental/economic integration that I believe is in the public interest.

CONFLICTING JURISDICTIONS AND THE DREADED ARARS

One of the biggest problems faced by those trying to site new waste-management facilities, or develop remediation programs for contaminated facilities, is the sheer number of regulations that may come into play. In 1994, then–EPA administrator Carol Browner was quoted as saying that the existing environmental regulatory scheme is "a complex and unwieldy system of laws and regulations [leading to] increasing conflict and gridlock."[12] The results of a 1993 survey published by the National Law Journal found that 70 percent of corporate environmental lawyers believed that full compliance with all municipal, state, and federal environmental laws was impossible.[13]

Environmental managers refer to this labyrinth of legal requirements as "the ARARs," an acronym for all *Applicable, Relevant, and Appropriate Regulations*. The ARARs include municipal regulations such as zoning restrictions, land use limitations, fire regulations, and the need for construction permits. They include state regulations on such issues as the transport of waste, the filing of drilling reports, and the disposal of contaminated soil. And they include federal regulations—the Clean Water Act and RCRA and the Superfund to be sure, but also labor regulations, antidiscrimination laws, tax laws, and maybe even laws relating to minority-owned businesses. There are so many of these laws that there are now computer databases on the market to allow environmental managers to search the entire body of federal and state law to cull out the applicable regulations. At one project with which I was involved, I recall seeing one of these computer-generated ARAR lists that ran to ten single-spaced pages.

In 1975, the total number of environmental regulations enacted over all time by all state and federal agencies and departments stood at about 2,000. By 1995, the list ran to more than 90,000.[14] A 1984 study by the Office of Technology Assessment of the U.S. Congress found that some aspects of groundwater contamination fell under fifteen different federal statutes involving twenty-four different federal agencies.[15] These agencies included the EPA and DOE of course, but also the Forest Service of the Department of Agriculture, the National Bureau of Standards of the Department of Commerce, the Bureau of Land Management and the National Parks Service of the Department of the Interior, and miscellaneous agencies of several other departments, including the Department of Defense and the Department of Transportation.

Sometimes these government agencies are in conflict with one another. It has been noted, for example, that 10 percent of the sites on the Superfund National Priorities List are federal facilities. Estimates of cleanup costs at major military bases run between $20 and $200 billion, and those at nuclear-weapons production facilities run to another $200 billion.[16] Current laws pit the EPA against the military, and against the DOE (which operates the nuclear weapons facilities). The various parties find themselves in a legal adversarial situation identical to that which exists between the EPA and corporate polluters. In many cases the adversarial situation leads to litigation. Surely, some type of integrated government policy could avoid these extended and costly intergovernmental litigations, thus saving huge amounts of public monies wasted in this internecine wrangling.

THE HEAVY HAND OF LEGISLATED STANDARDS

When the Superfund legislation was passed, it included a provision stating that the cleanup of contaminated sites should be carried out in compliance with all ARARs. Among the applicable, relevant, and appropriate regulations that then came into play were all the provisions of the Safe Drinking Water Act and its various amendments, including the maximum contaminant levels that had been established under this legislation for all the chemicals on the Priority Pollutants List. Because the MCLs are encoded in binding legislation, they have the weight of law. It is actually illegal to exceed them. By drafting the Superfund in the way they did, the legislators were in effect saying that they wanted all contaminated sites cleaned up to the level of the MCLs. As we have seen, this has not turned out to be technically or economically possible. Until the relatively recent arrival of the EPA's guidance on technical impracticability, regulators found themselves in the untenable position of either upholding the law and demanding a level of cleanup that was unattainable, or accepting something less and breaking the law. At almost every major Superfund site in the nation there have been endless rounds of heated discussion between the owner-operators of the sites demanding release from unreasonable standards and regulators explaining that under the law they are caught between a rock and a hard place. Even if they wanted to provide dispensation, they could not do so.

In most countries, environmental standards have the status of guidance rather than law. This allows regulators some leeway to negotiate realistic cleanup targets in special circumstances, and to develop consent orders with responsible parties that contain site-specific remediation targets. Most other countries have also recognized the intractability of drinking-water standards as cleanup targets at contaminated sites. In the Canadian provinces of Quebec and British Columbia, for example, a tiered system of cleanup standards has been established. It recognizes the difference between cleaning up a site for future residential use (and possible drinking-water development) and cleaning up a site to less demanding standards for future industrial use.

This discussion raises the more general issue of whether legislators should provide more or less flexibility in the legislation that they hand down to the regulatory agencies.[17] Lack of flexibility in U.S. regulations is based in part on congressional lack of trust in the regulatory agencies. It reflects public fears of power-crazed bureaucrats. The guiding rule is "Don't let the bureaucrats loose without precise instructions."[18] It is held that this more rigid approach lessens the opportunity for political interference and reduces the scope for legal adversarial proceedings. In my opinion, these supposed benefits of rigidity in regulation are outweighed by the need for flexibility to cope with site-specific complexities. There is a need to assess each site on its merits, taking into account site history, future use, potential risks, and economic and technical constraints. There is no question in my mind that the nondiscretionary use of drinking-water standards as targets for cleanup at contaminated sites in the Superfund program has led to unforgivable waste of public and private monies.

However, flexibility must not become an excuse for weakness. In most Canadian jurisdictions, where environmental guidelines rather than legislated standards are the norm, it can be argued that environmental protection has fallen far behind that achieved through the U.S. model. Government action tends to be driven by the media. Contaminated sites come to light only as a result of land transfer activities, not through systematic assessments of public risk. Long-term environmental planning is largely absent. Civil servants are overworked, and environmental agencies are understaffed. Clearly it is difficult to achieve the necessary balance between naked government power and a flexible regulatory milieu that is responsive to public needs.

Let us now turn to a more fundamental issue of regulatory policy. If we accept that environmental regulation involves setting standards, we must recognize that such standards may be one of two types: performance standards, or design standards.[19] Performance standards require that facilities achieve a certain level of performance without reference to how that performance is achieved. The Superfund program's reliance on achieving MCLs at specified compliance points fits into this regulatory philosophy. Design standards, on the other hand, require that facilities be constructed with specified methods and with certain design features. Much of the RCRA legislation fits into this regulatory framework, with its strict specification of the number of liners that must be included in landfills, its designation of acceptable leak-detection technologies, and its stipulation of specific monitoring-network strategies.

The argument against design standards is that they tend to cement in place outdated technologies and protocols. They do not encourage design innovation and are less responsive to new technical breakthroughs.

Performance standards would seem to be more straightforward. They allow design engineers their creative freedom but penalize them heavily if the facilities fail to perform. The problem here is that "failure" is not an immediate event. Compliance points where performance standards are checked and enforced are often some distance away from contaminant source areas, and migration rates may be quite slow. If penalties are not feared by owner-operators of waste-management facilities until sometime in the distant future, they may have little impact on current decisions and may not necessarily lead to the safe design and operation of the site in the near term. If penalties are too far in the future, a net-present-value economic analysis of current alternative designs or operational practices may discount them so significantly that they have little influence on current actions. From the regulatory perspective, the fines when they are collected may recoup the costs of enforcement and remediation, but they do not necessarily lead to facility designs that reduce risk to society.

It is hard to come down on one side or the other, and some mix of design standards and performance standards is probably good regulatory practice. In either case, however, it is imperative that sufficient flexibility be included to allow site-specific regulatory decision-making.

There is one last irony to report with respect to standards. In regional aquifers like those tapped in the San Gabriel and San Fernando basins of California, there are some portions of the aquifers that are contaminated with the solvent TCE, and some portions that are not. Prior to the promulgation of the MCL of 5 parts per billion for TCE, the great majority of people in these basins were receiving water with no TCE in it, but presumably a few were being served water with concentrations of TCE that exceeded the standard. One would assume that once the MCL became law, all the water-supply wells that were out of compliance would be shut down. Well, not quite. With the legal limit now established in black and white, some water companies who had both clean and dirty wells began blending the water from the two sets of wells, making sure to keep the concentrations of the blended water just under 5 parts per billion. The result was that almost all subscribers now received water with some TCE in it, even those who had previously received water that was completely free of TCE. In the past couple of years the EPA has taken steps against the blending of public water supplies, but the message to legislators and regulators seems clear. To every strategy there's a counterstrategy.

THE BIG STICK OF SUPERFUND

The Superfund has figured prominently in my discussions. It is time to look at it more closely. Its formal name is the Comprehensive Environmental Response, Compensation, and Liability Act (CERCLA). It was first passed in 1980, and it has been reauthorized several times since. It established a fund, fed by taxes on the chemical and petroleum industries, for the purpose of cleaning up contaminated sites. It has worked with a total annual budget of about $4 billion per year. The stated strategy is to clean up the sites first, and then litigate to recover the costs—the "shovels first, lawyers later" strategy.[20]

The Superfund has been a target for critics from its inception. It has been tabbed "superfailure" and "superfraud."[21] It has been brought to task by environmentalists for its failure to "clean up" sites and for its kowtowing to industry over the "technical impracticability" issue. It has been brought to task by industry over the cost of the cleanups, which often runs to tens of millions of dollars per site. And it has been criticized by all the parties over the pace of progress. With more than 1,200 sites on the National Priorities List, critics ask how it could be that five years into the program only 6 sites had been remediated, and after ten years only 41.[22] They note that the average time from inception to completion for all sites that have been completed to date has been on the order of twelve years.

Much of this criticism is unfair. The Superfund program has had to cope with a plethora of difficult problems. It has had to surmount unrealistic expectations, a shifting technical paradigm, and the environmental malaise of the Reagan era. While the pace of progress at individual sites must seem woefully slow to nontechnical observers, it must be said that the complexity of the undertaking is not understood by most of these observers. There are many steps in the remedial process at each site. They are all necessary and they all take time: (1) identification of the site, (2) preliminary assessment, (3) listing on the National Priorities List, if appropriate, (4) carrying out a remedial investigation to clarify site hydrogeology and determine the nature and extent of contamination, (5) carrying out a feasibility study and assessing potential remedial options, (6) negotiating a Record of Decision with the potentially responsible parties, (7) developing an engineering design for the selected remedial option, (8) constructing the remedial facility, and (9) bringing the remedial facility into operation. All this, while at the same time coping with ongoing negotiation, litigation, and public-relations activities with the owner-operator of the site, other potentially responsible parties, NIMBY groups, special-interest lobbyists, politicians, and press. Even the simple identification of potentially responsible parties (lovingly known as PRPs by EPA staff) can be a time-consuming, costly, and politically delicate task.

Statistics on the limited total number of remediated sites hide considerable progress in the other steps of the Superfund process. In the first ten years of the program, more than 28,000 sites were assessed, 1,200 were placed on the National Priorities List, 845 received remedial investigations and/or feasibility studies, and remediation was under way at 200 sites.[23] It must also be recognized that there are peripheral benefits.[24] The inventory of contaminated sites has value on its own. And there is no question that the Superfund jump-started the development of a site-restoration industry in the private sector. Perhaps the major achievement of the Superfund legislation was that it caused large corporations to take stock. They learned the hard way that the improper disposal of waste and the careless spillage of industrial chemicals would not be tolerated by society. They now know that the regulatory response will be swift and harsh. It can result in huge remedial and legal costs that have the potential to drive a company into bankruptcy.[25]

Without question, the most controversial element in the Superfund program is its system of liability. Prior to the Superfund, most liability systems applied to problems of public policy involved the establishment of fault, and compensation for harm done. The Superfund liability system is much harsher. It is based on the doctrines of absolute, retroactive, and joint-and-several liability. *Absolute liability* allows no defense of due diligence. Under this doctrine, owner-operators who cannot meet performance standards are liable for cleanup costs even if they can show that they used state-of-the-art methods and protocols in the operation of their facilities. *Retroactive liability* makes owner-operators liable even if the contamination occurred prior to the passage of the legislation, or prior to their ownership of the site. *Joint-and-several liability* holds that where there are many parties responsible for a contamination event, any one of them may be held liable for the total cost of cleanup of the entire site, without recourse to a fair-share allocation. It is based on the assumption that any PRP who feels unfairly treated will go to court to bring the other PRPs on board, thus shifting the cost of litigation from the public to the private purse.

To further complicate matters, Superfund PRPs are defined to include all past and present owners, operators, generators, and transporters of waste, and all are liable retroactively and jointly and severally. At the Stringfellow Acid Pits in California, for example, this included some 200 waste generators who sent waste to this facility in full compliance with the mandates of the state agency responsible at the time. At the OII Industries site in Monterey Park, California, it was estimated that there could be as many as 4,000 PRPs. A consent agreement involving 130 of them was finally negotiated as part of the Record of Decision.[26]

As noted by Thomas Church and Robert Nakamura in their book *Cleaning Up the Mess*, any doctrine that could hold someone who spills "a teacup of a mildly-toxic substance into a massive landfill" fully liable for all the expenses incident to its remediation, regardless of fault or negligence, and independent of any notion of fair-share allocation, requires some justification.[27] Clearly the potential for injustice is substantial. These authors suggest three rationales that might be put forward in defense of the Superfund liability doctrine. First, it may promote cooperative settlements among PRPs who want to avoid costly and time-consuming litigation (the *settlement rationale*). Second, it gives the EPA the leverage to force rich corporations to pay for cleanups (the *deep pockets rationale*). And third, it is expected to be a positive influence on the future behavior of corporate America (the *incentive rationale*).

Unfortunately these rationales, especially the one suggesting that cooperative settlements would emerge, were not prescient. Instead, corporate America simply got its back up. The patent unfairness of the liability provisions provoked resistance and obstruction on the part of the PRPs. Sites bogged down in legal wrangling, and owner-operators developed a cynical disdain for the regulatory process. They found it cheaper and more satisfying to pay lawyers to litigate rather than engineers to remediate.

As individuals, most of us would feel extremely ill treated if penalized for something that is illegal now but wasn't when we did it, particularly if it was common practice at the time. Representatives of the waste-generating industries feel the same. The loss of goodwill between industry and regulators over the retroactivity clause may outweigh the value of any cost recovery that has been achieved. It is unlikely that cooperative compliance can be achieved in the climate of mutual suspicion that has been generated by the Superfund liability provisions. It is likely that the Superfund would have worked better had it put away the big stick and tried to use a softer and fairer doctrine of liability.

From the beginning, the Superfund has been plagued with two major issues: How clean is clean enough? And who should pay, and how do we make them do so? Critics argue that by setting unrealistic compliance targets, the Superfund created technical gridlock; and by setting unfair liability provisions, it created legal gridlock. Supporters claim that without these provisions nothing would have been done. In retrospect, it appears that the early policies may have indeed been too rigid. In recent years the environmental pendulum has swung back toward policies that may be less satisfying to environmentalists but are probably based on more achievable objectives. It is hard to satisfy everyone. The controversy rages on, with one side claiming that not enough is being accomplished, and the other side claiming that too much money is being wasted and the dollars would be better spent elsewhere. It is not likely to subside soon.

THE RED HERRING OF COST RECOVERY

Every environmental cleanup law that has ever been written includes legal procedures for the recovery of cleanup costs from those parties that caused the pollution. Every politician who stands up to defend an environmental bill is almost sure to emphasize that the bill is based on the principle of "polluter pays." The funding of the Superfund cleanup program, for example, comes not only from the tax on chemical feedstocks that creates the fund but also on direct recovery of costs from responsible parties at contaminated sites. The corporations publicly announce the vast sums that they are spending on cleanup; the politicians crow that the companies are getting their just desserts; and the public takes it all in at face value.

There is only one problem. It is not really true. Publicly owned companies cannot easily swallow expenditures of this size without concern for the rest of their balance sheet. They have shareholders to please, profit margins to meet, and stock prices that must be defended. They simply pass their environmental costs on to the consumer. They do so through increased prices for the goods they produce. The costs of environmental cleanup are not borne by the polluters; they are borne by you and me.

If one looks at the financing details at a contaminated site, one usually finds that the funds for environmental cleanup come from three pots: corporate accounts, government coffers, and the insurance industry. These are the economic entities that sign the checks. But in all three cases, the real source of the funds is the individual citizens of the nation. We pay for environmental cleanup through increased consumer prices, increased taxation, and increased insurance premiums. The costs of environmental cleanup are social costs. They are borne by society at large, and there is really no way around it.

It is likely that politicians who include cost recovery provisions in environmental legislation are fully aware that these costs are passed on to the consumer, but the public has been slower to appreciate this fact, and for the politicians the appearance of putting it to the corporations is a political currency too valuable to throw away. Environmentalists have been frustrated for years over this issue. They feel that the guilty parties are somehow slipping away in the night without getting their proper comeuppance. Their desire for more personal accountability has led them to push for criminal prosecution of individual corporate officers in cases of environmental degradation. While this might be appropriate for future corporate transgressions of current environmental law, I find it a difficult strategy to support in cases of historical contamination, where malicious intent is unlikely.

Unfortunately, if the public is not more cognizant of who really pays for environmental cleanup, then it is little inclined to weigh the benefits of cleanup against the costs, thinking that the costs are truly being borne by the corporations. The result is a lack of public concern over the social costs of environmental overkill. The media have not been helpful in this regard. They have shown little interest in providing in-depth coverage of environmental issues, preferring to push the public's hot buttons with continuing tales of toxic terror.

The current method of cost recovery almost guarantees an unpleasant and inefficient adversarial climate. As a result, a large portion of program expenditures now goes not to remedial actions but to transaction costs—fees for lawyers and technical consultants who support the warring factions in their conflicts over the allocation of responsibility and the recovery of costs. These transaction costs could be much reduced if politicians and regulators could see their way clear to creating a more cooperative environment for negotiated settlements among the parties.

The arguments of this section should not be seen as a plea to release the polluting industries from their responsibilities. Now that the situation is clear, with the causes and effects of careless waste-handling practices understood, corporations must be held accountable for the development of proper protocols of preventive practice, and for transgressions against such practice, should they occur. The cleanup of historical contamination, on the other hand, could be accomplished more effectively if the goal were the minimization of the overall social cost, rather than the assignment of blame and the recovery of costs through adversarial litigation.

ENVIRONMENTAL MORALITY

There is a touchy subject lurking in the wings of the debate over environmental regulation. It is the question of morality, and the role of punishment for environmental misdeeds. Certainly, if you or I were to go out right now in full knowledge of a particular environmental statute and willfully break the law, then there would be no question that what we had done was immoral (as well as illegal), and that we ought to be punished. More realistically, perhaps, if some type of collusion can be proven between a corporate management team and individual employees to violate environmental laws, then both the company and the individuals should be liable to prosecution.

Most culpable actions of this type are addressed in the criminal provisions in the laws of the land. Environmental violations can be met by administrative action, by civil fines, or by criminal prosecution. The situation becomes fuzzier when we begin to consider some of the responsible parties caught in the Superfund net. It is hard to ascribe immoral motives to waste generators who disposed of waste in a responsible fashion under the protocols of the day but who have now become miscreants under the retroactivity doctrines of the Superfund. Perhaps it is for this reason that there are no direct punishment provisions in the Superfund statutory framework.[28] The legislators may have recognized that the cleanup of historical contamination is not about moral rights and wrongs: it is a practical matter of protecting human health. As a counterexample, in the RCRA legislation, which deals largely with the construction and operation of *new* waste-management facilities, failure to meet the regs is viewed as arising out of malice aforethought. RCRA spells out clear penalties for environmental violations.

The lack of a moral underpinning to the Superfund program would be well and good were it not for the contrary views held by many individual regulators. In their eyes, environmental degradation *is* a moral crime and those responsible deserve punishment. When the law was passed, the failure to include punitive provisions did not particularly upset this constituency because they assumed (along with many of the legislators, I suspect) that the cleanup costs would directly reflect the level of carelessness and maliciousness on the part of the responsible parties. They assumed that the worst actors would pay the heaviest price. This has not turned out to be the case. Their assumption failed to take into account the diversity of settings of contaminated sites, the differing nature of their hydrogeological environments, and the wide spectrum of offsite contaminant migration rates. Some PRPs are lucky and some are unlucky. The lucky ones fortuitously discover that their site contamination has little impact on the surrounding environment, and that a minimal remedial program will set things right. The unlucky ones discover that a minor slipup in their waste-management practices has led to the regional contamination of a major drinking-water aquifer, and it will cost millions to set it right.

As an example of good luck, take the Kodak plant in Rochester, New York. This is a huge facility with a long history and many documented solvent releases over the years. However, through good fortune, it turns out that the Kodak site is underlain by relatively low-permeability rocks, there is no significant discharge of contaminants to any surface-water bodies, and there are no aquifers beneath the site. In fact, not only are there no aquifers present, but the groundwater itself is too saline to drink in any case. The contaminants enter a groundwater flow system that is flowing at Rip van Winkle rates and is not a viable resource in the first place. To cap it all off, there is a network of storm water drainage tunnels ringing the site that was constructed by the municipality for different purposes but which now serves as an almost perfectly designed hydraulic control on any offsite migration that might occur.

Contrast the Kodak story with that of the Elf-Atochem site in Tacoma, Washington, where the arsenic-based herbicide penite was manufactured, as described in chapter 2. The Elf-Atochem site is a very small facility covering only a few acres, with a source of arsenic contamination of limited size. The volume of material causing the problem is orders of magnitude smaller than that on the Kodak site. As fate would have it, however, the Elf-Atochem site sits on the banks of the Hylebos Waterway, a part of the Commencement Bay Superfund site. The soils underlying the site are high-permeability sands that drain directly into the Hylebos. In addition, there are complex geochemical effects that make the arsenic more mobile than it would otherwise be.[29] To compound the bad luck, it turns out that arsenic is particularly harmful to the marine biota that populate Commencement Bay.

At the Elf-Atochem facility, huge expenditures have been required, which even regulatory officials see as being out of proportion to the size of the site and the nature of the contamination. At the Kodak site, where the necessity of cleaning up the historical contamination cannot really be defended, I sense that regulators are frustrated by their inability to punish Kodak for its past actions. (It is only fair to point out that Kodak's historical practices were no better and no worse than those of other large corporations of the day, and that their response to environmental pressures in recent years has been cooperative and proactive. In addition, they have spent considerable sums on preventive measures under RCRA.)

There is no question that the lack of moral compass creates a conundrum for the regulators involved in the day-to-day enforcement of environmental legislation. They face a full spectrum of corporate responses to their regulatory pressure, from proactive cooperation to cynical disdain. They would like to go easy on the good guys and throw the book at the bad guys, but the facts don't always fit their wishes. I have been involved in a couple of projects where the temptations for regulatory revenge put the agencies in technically indefensible positions and led to protracted legal conflict that served no good purpose. In these situations it must be hard to watch the bad guys getting away without a good hiding. On the other side of the coin, my heart goes out to the many small, almost-innocent, mom-and-pop operations that get entangled in large Superfund settlements. It is sometimes difficult to accept that the goal is the minimization of public health risk, not the adjudication of moral rights and wrongs.

ENVIRONMENTAL JUSTICE

As I noted earlier, environmental regulation, like all regulation, leaves winners and losers in its wake. An assessment of environmental justice seeks to identify these winners and losers to see if the distribution is in some sense "just."

In the regulatory framework that has grown up to control waste-management strategies and reduce environmental contamination, the suite of winners is very large, encompassing every citizen who benefits from any reduction in health risk that may be achieved. The suite of losers is much smaller, but it could be argued that the losses they are asked to bear can be quite substantial. They are the citizens who are asked to bear the loss in property values and possible added risk that come with hosting a waste-management facility in their community. It will probably not come as much of a surprise to learn who these losers are. In a democratic society the losers tend to be those who are politically weak, and in a capitalist society those who are politically weak are those who are economically weak. In short, those who are least well-off will be asked to bear the brunt of the additional risks associated with environmental regulation.

Studies have shown that there are more waste-management facilities in poor communities than in communities that are better off. A study carried out in Los Angeles County identified eighty-two hazardous-waste treatment, storage, and disposal facilities in the county.[30] Correlations were attempted between the location of these facilities and several demographic variables including per capita income, median home value, level of unemployment, percentage of residents with high school education, percentage of residents registered to vote, and percentage of minority residents (African American, Asian, Hispanic, and Native American). The results show substantial demographic inequity. In short, "the communities that are likely to host a facility are neighborhoods with a large concentration of working-class people of color." Perhaps even more disturbing is the fact that the correlations for racial-ethnic indicators are even clearer than those for economic indicators.

With so many more contaminated sites on the poor side of town than on the rich side, one would assume that a larger number of cleanups under Superfund and/or state remediation programs would also take place there. Not so. It turns out that despite the smaller number of sites on the well-off side of town, more cleanups take place there than on the poor side.[31] It seems clear that money talks. Those on the rich side of town have the money to spend to get organized and get their point of view heard. They have the education and the expertise to assess the issues and understand the workings of the system. They may also have better political connections.

The pessimistic conclusion of this section is that the results of environmental regulation do not necessarily lead to social justice. More likely, the indirect income redistribution produced by environmental regulation enriches the rich and impoverishes the poor.

THE NEED FOR PRIORITIZATION

The allocation of public monies is a thankless task. Liberals demand the redistribution of wealth from the advantaged to the disadvantaged. Conservatives demand tax cuts and subsidies for industry to allow them to go about their business of creating jobs and generating wealth. Elections over these issues are won or lost by 51 percent to 49 percent. Consensus is never achieved.

The allocation of monies that is ordained by environmental laws suffers the same lack of consensus. Priorities are never met with universal approval. Environmentalists fume, "Too little." The new right fumes, "Too much." One of the few items of consensus that comes through this cacophony of value-laden rhetoric is the feeling that environmental expenditures, regardless of whether they are large or small, ought to be carefully prioritized. Everyone seems to agree that environmental monies earmarked for the protection of human health ought to be spent where the greatest reduction in health risk can be achieved for the fewest dollars.

As we have seen, this does not always happen. When regulations arise through the desire to quell short-term public alarm over environmental accidents, missed connections abound, costs and benefits are seldom in concert, and the dollars spent per life saved vary widely across the suite of risk-reducing regulations. There is a clear need for an improvement in the prioritization process. This is true not only within the Superfund program but also across the full suite of environmental programs and strategies, and between environmental expenditures and those for other social programs.

Within the Superfund program, there is little evidence that the National Priorities List (NPL) bears any great reciprocity to actual site risks across the nation.[32] One would assume that sites would be prioritized by the degree of risk to public health, the need to act quickly to control contamination, the feasibility of engineered solutions, and the likelihood of achieving remedial goals with low-cost technologies. Unfortunately the NPL listings have followed a much more political course. The distribution of Superfund sites is much more consistent with "the political objective of obtaining a high level of congressional support"[33] than it is with remedial needs. Certainly, the most threatening sites in the nation *are* on the list, and there *are* more sites on the list from industrial states like New York and New Jersey than from less populated, agrarian, midwestern states like Nebraska or Wyoming. Still, the list shows unmistakable political influence: states without any real problem sites still get their share, and almost every congressional district has at least one site on the list.

An example from my own experience tells the tale. A few years ago I found myself working as a consultant on two Superfund sites at the same time: the Lowry landfill in Denver, Colorado, and the San Fernando groundwater basin near Los Angeles, California. Contamination in the San Fernando Valley threatens the drinking-water supply of a million people; the limited surficial contamination at the Lowry landfill doesn't threaten anyone's drinking-water supply. Yet under the congressional pork-barreling of the day, the two sites were funded at roughly the same level.

When it comes to the broader question of environmental programs and strategies, there are a variety of prioritization issues that ought to be examined. We need to decide whether environmental expenditures should be allocated (1) to favor the cleanup of historical contamination or the prevention of future contamination; (2) to support construction and operation of new pollution control facilities or the monitoring, performance assessment, and enforcement of regulatory compliance at existing facilities; (3) to achieve water pollution reduction or air pollution reduction; (4) to address human health risk reduction or ecological habitat protection; and (5) to control individual contaminated sites or attend to environmental questions of larger global import like ozone depletion and global warming.

I spoke earlier of the advantages of prevention over remediation as a policy alternative. There is a need to see higher priority given to the preventive policy instruments discussed in chapter 4: watershed management initiatives, land use restrictions, wellhead protection strategies, and the sole-source aquifer program.[34] I believe that cost-benefit studies based on a risk-management approach would lead to greater use of these preventive administrative controls in place of the widespread current use of engineered remedial controls.

Most of these preventive approaches to environmental protection take place at the scale of aquifers and watersheds rather than that of individual contaminated sites. However, there is a connection. In addition to their preventive goals, regional studies identify sensitive wetlands, aquifers, and recharge areas, and the presence or absence of these features ought to be an important element in setting priorities on contaminated sites for remediation.

One lesson learned in almost all jurisdictions is that it is much easier to legislate environmental regulations than to enforce them once they are in place. The cost of enforcement has been systematically underestimated in almost all regulatory programs designed to protect the environment. One study has suggested that as many as 25 percent of all water utilities in the United States are out of compliance with EPA standards.[35] The states often abdicate the enforcement responsibilities that have been passed on to them by the EPA, and the EPA doesn't have the money or staff to enforce its own laws. If our environmental laws are to be effective, it is likely that funds will have to be redirected from the more proactive aspects of the legislated programs into the enforcement sector.

The balance between water pollution expenditures and air pollution expenditures has long been a bone of contention in environmental circles. Studies both internal and external to the EPA suggest that current priorities do not reflect the relative risks.[36] It is estimated that by the year 2000 the nation's total pollution control costs will run to $160 billion per year, with water pollution costs running about two to one over air pollution costs.[37] A study by the Natural Resources Defense Council claims that the average life expectancy in major American cities is reduced by one to three years due to lung and heart problems aggravated by urban air pollution. Air pollution controls thus have the potential to produce a statistically significant increase in life expectancy for a large number of Americans. No such widespread health impact can be claimed for the water pollution prevention achieved by contaminated-sites regulations such as the Superfund and RCRA.

Most observers also feel that global-scale environmental questions are underfunded. Clearly the potential risks to humankind as a whole from atmospheric ozone depletion, global warming, and climate change are much greater than the risks that accrue to those few people unfortunate enough to live near a contaminated site. The level of the global risk is still uncertain, but surely the threat is sufficiently great to warrant the necessary level of scientific activity to reduce the uncertainty. On the basis of the most recent studies, it seems clear that the cancer risk associated with depletion of the atmospheric ozone layer, if such depletion is confirmed, is much greater than that associated with the presence of contaminated sites.

This argument is not meant to belittle the fears of those who live near contaminated sites, but as we have seen in earlier chapters, the actual risks are much lower than the perceived risks, and the actual risks can be successfully reduced with much less costly programs than we are currently supporting with our tax dollars. Some of the money saved by correcting the overkill in dealing with environmental contamination could profitably be redirected to correcting the underkill on these global environmental issues.

What about the total context of environmental expenditures? Do we have reason to question the prioritization of government expenditures on the environment vis-à-vis those earmarked for other social programs? Arguments can certainly be made in this direction. On the health front alone, there are apparent gross inequities between programs. In 1993, the Superfund was allocated $1.75 billion in public monies to address the EPA's estimate of 1,000 cancer cases per year arising from hazardous-waste contamination. In the same year, breast cancer programs were allocated one thousand times less ($133 million) to address the 175,000 cases of breast cancer that arise each year.[38] That's $1.75 million per cancer case for environmental contamination, and less than $1,000 per case for breast cancer. Something is amiss.

If we let ourselves rove even more widely through the social net, we must surely come to the tragic conditions of inner-city poverty. As a Canadian, I am flabbergasted by the apparent lack of interest during American presidential elections in this inner-city decay. As an election issue it doesn't even make the top ten list in *Time* and *Newsweek*. The poverty and despair of the people trapped in city slums cries out for compassion. If America is willing to put remediation of the Love Canal onto its top priority list, why not the remediation of our inner cities? When it comes to national health and happiness, there is no question in my mind which problem poses the greater threat. There is evidence here of selfishness in the allocation of public priorities. Surely there must also be priorities of the heart.

There will be those who will try to use some of these arguments to support a reduction of the overall tax load on American citizens. That would be a misreading of my case. Many other countries, Canada among them, sustain a stronger social net through higher rates of taxation than those assessed in the United States. In my opinion, the U.S. social net is inadequate, especially as it relates to inner-city poverty. I am espousing more careful prioritization of public monies across the full suite of government programs. I believe that there is scope for redirection of resources between programs within the environmental framework, and between environmental programs and the wider net of nonenvironmental social programs. I do not support reduction of the overall tax load; on the contrary, current tax rates may be inadequate to cope with the various threats to the nation's health, environmental and otherwise.

THE BOTTOM LINE

- There will always be need for a strong regulatory presence in matters of environmental protection. We need regulations that provide sufficient protection of the environment but do not waste valuable societal resources that would be better spent elsewhere. Current contaminated-sites legislation has created conditions of over-regulation that are not in the public interest. However, current thrusts toward deregulation have become too ideological. What is needed now is not repeal but fine-tuning.

- The case for regulatory rationalization revolves around five issues: (1) the need to reevaluate the Priority Pollutants List, with an eye to removing some of the more benign toxicants from it; (2) the need to relax the maximum contaminant levels for many chemicals; (3) the need to replace MCL-driven cleanups at contaminated sites with risk-based decision processes; (4) the need to bring acceptable-risk levels in environmental matters into balance with the risk levels accepted in other walks of life; and (5) the need to move from source-area restoration technologies toward containment technologies that protect drinking-water aquifers from contamination.

- There are so many environmental regulations now in place, and so many different agencies administering them, that full compliance with all municipal, state, and federal laws may well be impossible. The lack of integration across regulatory programs often leads to inconsistent compliance requirements and unintended environmental consequences. Recent initiatives designed to address the "brownfields syndrome" provide an encouraging model of environmental/economic integration that is in the public interest.

- There is a need for flexibility in environmental regulations that allows regulatory personnel to cope with site-specific complexities. The rigid use of drinking-water standards as compliance targets for cleanup at contaminated industrial sites in the Superfund program has led to an unacceptable waste of public and private monies.

- The lack of moral justice in the retroactive and joint-and-several liability provisions in the Superfund legislation has provoked resistance and obstruction on the part of potentially responsible parties at contaminated sites. The detrimental effects of the resulting legal gridlock outweigh the value of any added cost recovery that has been achieved through the application of these liability doctrines. It is likely that the Superfund would be more successful in gaining cooperative settlements were it to use a softer and fairer doctrine of liability.

- The administration of current environmental regulations does not necessarily lead to social justice. The great majority of all waste-management facilities are located in communities with large concentrations of working-class people of color. Yet, despite the smaller number of sites in well-off communities, more remedial cleanups take place there than in poorer communities.

- There are opportunities for redirecting priorities between programs within the existing suite of environmental strategies. Environmental expenditures should be allocated in a way that assigns higher priority to preventing future contamination than to remediating historical contamination, to reducing air pollution than to reducing water pollution, and to addressing questions of larger global impact like ozone depletion and global warming than to controlling individual contaminated sites.

- There is also scope for redirecting resources from the environmental sector as a whole toward the solution of social problems, such as inner-city poverty, that pose a greater threat to the health and happiness of the nation.

• These arguments do not support a reduction of the overall tax load. Current U.S. tax rates are lower than those in many other developed countries and may be inadequate to cope with the various threats to the nation's health, environmental and otherwise.

7 The Environmental Game

The environmental game is a game in the same sense that war is a game. Environmental decisions take place in an atmosphere of conflict. There are many players and ample opportunity for tactical alliances, collusion, and betrayal. Thankfully there are fewer lives at stake, but as in a real war, while the fight may appear to be over ideology, it is often also about money and turf. As in a real war, it is a zero-sum game. There are winners and losers; one party's loss is another party's gain. To the winners go the spoils.

SWINGING ON THE PENDULUM: THE PLAYERS
IN THE ENVIRONMENTAL GAME

In Table 18 we see the players at the ready: the rule makers, the PRPs, those drawn into the fray, those feeding at the trough, and those stirring the pot. It is a complex mix, and it doesn't make for easy negotiations or quick settlements. It is politics with a small "p." There is lots of room for entrenched positions, personality conflicts, and frustrated emotions.

The politicians see the environmental game as a lose/lose situation. They are pressured by the environmentalists to pass legislation that puts it to the corporations and gets contaminated sites cleaned up better and faster. They are pressured by the corporations and the insurance companies to go slower, reduce the Superfund taxes, and soften the liability doctrines. They are pressured by the technical community to get a better handle on the health effects, and to await improvements in restoration technologies, before setting up regulations that are carved in stone. And they are pressured by individual constituents to get cracking on the cleanup of local sites. No wonder they have developed their own version of NIMBY. It's known as NIMTO—Not In My Term of Office.

The regulators have their own problems. They are the most powerful players in the game, yet they are often undertrained and understaffed. The usual career path for an environmental scientist these days is to hire on with the EPA or a state agency right out of school, learn the ropes on a government salary, then jump to a more lucrative position in the consulting industry when the opportunity arises. The consulting companies, who serve the waste generators for the most part, get to watch these young scientists and engineers in action during the technical negotiations that accompany every cleanup. They pluck the good ones up and leave the less talented to truck on with the agencies. Of course, there are some very talented regulatory personnel who don't jump—the ones who are most committed to the environmental ethic, and those who don't want to risk becoming apologists for bad guys. Nevertheless there is a filter in operation here that tends to lead to an uneven distribution of talent between industry and the regulatory agencies. If we view the fundamental environmental conflict as one between the waste-generating

Table 18 The players in the environmental game.

Rulemakers	Public
	Politicians/legislators
	Regulatory agencies
Potentially responsible parties (PRPs)	Owner/operators of waste facilities
	Corporate waste generators: the chemical and petroleum industry
	Government waste generators: the DOE and the military
	Insurance companies
Drawn into the fray	Host communities
	Mom-and-pop PRPs
Feeding at the trough	Lawyers
	Technical consultants/expert witnesses
	Cleanup industry
Stirring the pot	Environmentalists
	NIMBY groups
	Interested spectators: professional organizations, service clubs, labor unions, university research laboratories
	Media

firms, who contribute to the economic health of society, and government regulatory agencies, who protect societal interests with respect to health and the environment, then it is important to society that the two sides be evenly matched. In the long run, an unequal adversarial process will lead to poor-quality decision-making and a potential for environmental underprotection. To stem the current brain drain from government service into the private sector, it is necessary that the regulatory agencies keep their salary structure competitive with that of industry and provide a creative and challenging workplace for their most talented technical people.

The potentially responsible parties come in all shades: the good, the bad, and the ugly. In my consulting life, I have seen the full gamut, from the proactive cooperation of Union Pacific, Elf-Atochem, and Ciba-Geigy at their sites in Laramie, Wyoming; Tacoma, Washington; and Toms River, New Jersey, to the legal and technical hardball of several of the PRPs in the San Fernando basin. Most major American corporations— the Lockheeds, the Kodaks, and the IBMs—have developed a pragmatic, if uneasy, working relationship with the regulators. They still feel that they are being asked to bear an unfair share of the burden, and they still rail against the unfair liability provisions of the Superfund, but they are big enough to weather the blows, and after twenty years of futile skirmishing they are now more or less on board. It is the mid-size companies that have the biggest problems. They have sufficiently deep pockets to attract the attention of the regulators, but they worry that the imposition of these huge, unexpected environmental expenditures could take away whatever competitive advantages they enjoy in their marketplace, or even drive them to bankruptcy. These are the companies most likely to hire a stonewalling lawyer and move to new premises.

The insurance companies are a special case. They carry the environmental liability policies of the PRPs, and in a sense they become PRPs themselves. When the first regulatory enforcement actions hit the fan back in the early eighties, the insurance companies were caught off guard. They found themselves ensnared in a web of litigation and potential liability that limited their ability to underwrite insurance. They worried that it might ultimately threaten their financial viability.[1] To borrow from a recent country western song, the insurance reps took on the role of "Cleopatra, Queen of Denial," denying that their clients were responsible, denying that their policies provided coverage, or denying that contamination occurred during the periods covered by their policies. Almost all of the cases that ended up in court in the early years were "Who pays?" cases, and the great majority of these were insurance cases. I know that my phone rang off the hook in those days, as insurance lawyers tried to round up expert witnesses who would testify as to the exact dates that a contamination incident started and stopped, trying to prove that *their* policies were not in effect at the time. I gave a wide berth to these unsavory cases. Having learned what it was worth, I also canceled my liability insurance.

The host communities of contaminated sites or prospective waste-management facilities often feel powerless to control their own destiny. Their municipal mandates are superseded by the powerful state and federal statutes. Their limited technical expertise is overwhelmed by the lawyers, consultants, and technical experts who descend on their town. They are limited to an intervenor role in the negotiation process that accompanies the siting of new facilities or the restoration of old ones, just one voice in the many that have a right to be heard. They find their communities being used as a stage for the ideological battles over environmental policy.

The beneficiaries of the environmental game are the lawyers, consultants, and expert witnesses who are hired to provide legal and technical support to the parties in conflict, and the burgeoning cleanup industry, which gets to carry out research and development programs with paying customers. Life is so good for consultants in New Jersey that the Environmental Cleanup and Responsibility Act (ECRA) is locally referred to as the Environmental Consultants Retirement Act.[2] On the cleanup front, an advertisement recently crossed my desk asking me to subscribe to a weekly newsletter called *Defense Cleanup*. Published "from offices near the Pentagon" it suggested that I "follow the $$$ trail" by getting my piece of the $24 billion dollars currently in the Defense Environmental Restoration Account, or the $400 billion expected to be spent by DOE in the next decade for the restoration of the old weapons facilities across the nation. For just $395 per year, it promised to tell me how to hit this jackpot.

Finally, ringing the playing field and waiting their turn to get into the action are the interested spectators, pinch hitters, and downfield tacklers—the environmental groups, with a long and honorable history but zero tolerance for compromise; the NIMBY groups, who often ride on the environmentalists' coattails but have a much simpler agenda; the professional organizations, service clubs, labor unions, and university research labs; and of course, the press, stirring the pot with rumors and innuendo, looking for the big story.

The environmental game is played according to the rules laid down in whatever environmental statute is brought to bear on the problem. Like a baseball game, there are many innings, and each team gets many turns at bat. Recall the many steps in the Superfund process: listing on the National Priorities List (the NPL), remedial investigations, feasibility studies, a Record of Decision, and design and operation of the remedial facility. At each step in the proceedings there are only a certain number of alternative courses of action on the table, and all the players in the game undoubtedly know which course of action they would most like to see. In addition, they can probably rank the rest of the options in order of acceptability from their perspective (their *preference vectors*, in the jargon of the day). The EPA and the NIMBY groups will want to see a contaminated site listed on the NPL so that the heavy hammer of the Superfund can be brought into play; the PRPs and the insurance companies will undoubtedly prefer that the site not be listed. Usually the preferred remedial option for a given party is the one that will attain all of their goals at no cost to themselves. The EPA will prefer a total cleanup, funded fully by the PRPs; the PRPs will prefer no cleanup at all, or limited cleanup funded from governmental coffers. The EPA will seek to recover its costs; the PRPs will resist.

At each stage of the proceedings, a decision must be made. Will the site be listed on the NPL or not? What remedial action will be approved in the Record of Decision? Who will pay for it, and how much? The decisions that are reached at these decision points can arise in one of several ways.[3] They can be unilaterally handed down by the regulatory agency under the authority vested in it by the statutes, in which case the PRPs may get their backs up and go into delay-and-stonewall mode. They can arise from negotiation among the parties, which would seem to be the most desirable route. Or they can come from judicial decisions handed down in a court of law as a result of litigation between the parties. The options that have some chance of surviving a negotiated or judicial settlement usually lie well down on the preference vectors of all the parties. They will be compromise positions that leave none of the parties entirely happy.

At each stage of the proceedings, all the players in the game require technical information to back up their position, and legal representation to advance their position through the negotiation or judicial process. The major players usually find it necessary to hire two support teams, one an engineering consulting firm to advance their technical objectives, and the other a law firm to advance their legal objectives. The number of players in the game is thus multiplied by three at a single stroke. In insurance cases, it is multiplied manyfold, because the insurance carriers never shoulder all the risk themselves. They lay some of it onto other insurance companies, each of which will want its own technical and legal teams to protect its interests. I recall attending a meeting in Los Angeles of the PRPs who had been identified by the EPA as candidates for cost recovery under the Superfund remedial program in the San Fernando basin. There were at least twenty technical consultants in the room, and more than fifty lawyers representing the interests of the various participants. In a talk at a recent environmental conference, Marcel Moreau, a regulator with the Maine Department of Environmental Protection, put the situation succinctly: "There is a fundamental conflict between American business and environmental regulations that can never be resolved. When both regulator and businessman are doing their job this conflict is inevitable. Under the circumstances, we need to keep our perspective and our sense of humor."[4]

Some environmental games are unfair (like ticktacktoe, where whoever goes first wins). Some are like the Prisoner's Dilemma, where there is no optimal solution. And in the eyes of some of the players, there are parallels with the military doomsday scenarios of the fifties, which seemed to imply that the optimal strategy under some circumstances was to blow up the world. To some degree, the more powerful parties can impose their will on the weaker parties, moving negotiated settlements farther up their own preference vectors at the expense of the preferences of their adversaries. There is no question that in the 1970s and 1980s the government regulatory agencies claimed the most powerful negotiating position, with the full support of the public and the big stick of the Superfund as their bequest from the legislators to carry out the public will. As we have seen, the results were a mixture of progress and frustration, with a large component of technical and economic gridlock.

As we come to the turn of the century, we are seeing a change in the power structure, a willingness to consider more options, and a softening of attitudes toward the preference vectors of adversarial parties. There is reason for optimism. There is potential in the coming years for a more cooperative perspective among the parties, based on a softer, more balanced, and participatory approach to negotiation, and less reliance on legal adversarial conflict.[5]

If this era of more enlightened environmental decision-making is to come to pass, we must avoid repeating the mistakes of the past. In the sections that follow, we will look at many of the issues that require the attention of decision makers: the recognition of technical uncertainty, the avoidance of social bias, and the need for better integration of the technical and legal search for truth. It will be necessary to step back from divisive and unfair policies of cost recovery, and insure that legal gridlock does not delay the necessary preventive actions.

ROADBLOCKS TO CONSENSUS: TECHNICAL UNCERTAINTY AND SOCIAL BIAS

A few years ago I found myself sitting in the witness box as an expert witness in a court case involving the adjudication of costs between two parties in an environmental lawsuit. The legal team on each side had hired technical consultants, of which I was one, to back up their claim that their client was not responsible for the remedial costs incurred. Each of the technical teams had scoured the available data, developed their interpretations of site conditions, and plugged into the latest computer models to bolster their interpretation. I went into the lawsuit assuming that the two technical interpretations would look pretty much the same. Not so. The results were startlingly different. And in each case, the engineering interpretations put forward by the technical witnesses strongly supported the legal claims of their own client.

Now this may not come as any great surprise to the reader, but I must admit that it was a great surprise to me at the time. As an engineer, I had always been led to believe that technical information was value-free, and that given the same information, two technical teams—assuming both were honest and ethical—would come to the same conclusion. In the case at hand, I felt that the team of which I was a member had been scrupulously objective in reaching conclusions. I was also familiar with the technical team that represented our adversaries, and I knew them to be an honest and ethical firm.

In the court case, after I had given my evidence and been cross-examined by the lawyers for the other side, the judge asked me a few questions himself. One of them was, "How can two reputable technical firms, looking at the same data, have come to such diametrically opposite conclusions?" I must admit that at the time I was just as flabbergasted as he was, and my answer was probably not very satisfactory. Since then, I have seen the same situation time and again, and I have given more thought to how it comes to pass. I now believe that there are two contributing factors. One is the presence of technical uncertainty in environmental studies, and the other is what I will call social bias. These two factors act as roadblocks to consensus, both in the court cases themselves and in attempts to reach out-of-court, negotiated settlements.

Let us look at each of these issues in turn.

No matter how much site characterization is carried out during the remedial investigation at a contaminated site, there is always some level of technical uncertainty that remains. Each hole drilled at the site, each chemical analysis of a sample of soil or water from the site, in fact, each and every step in the site characterization program, serves to reduce the uncertainty about the nature of the hydrogeological environment at the site, the nature and extent of contamination, and the fate and transport of the contaminants. However, this process of uncertainty reduction is never complete. The geologists are always begging to drill one more hole; the engineers are always demanding one more test. Eventually the site manager decides that enough is enough. There comes a time when in that person's judgment the costs of further investigation outweigh the likely benefits. But uncertainty still remains, and this uncertainty is the prism through which a rainbow of alternative interpretations can survive.

Table 19 outlines the breadth of technical uncertainty that can arise

Table 19 Some sources of technical uncertainty.

Data	Accuracy of measured parameters
	Representativeness of measured parameters
	Worth of additional data
Interpretation of the data	Interpretation of geological environment
	Interpretation of groundwater flow system
	Interpretation of extent of contaminant plume
Physical and chemical processes	Nature of contaminants and their properties
	Processes and rates of contaminant migration
Performance of engineered remediation	Effectiveness of contaminant removal technologies such as bioreclamation or surfactant flushing

in environmental disputes at a contaminated site. There are uncertainties over data, over the interpretations of the data, over the contaminant migration processes that are important at the site, and over the engineering performance that can be expected from proposed remedial actions.

Let's look at just a couple of the issues listed in Table 19. Take the question of the accuracy of measured chemical analyses on groundwater samples that have been collected at a site. Chemical sampling and analysis have become expensive and highly specialized operations. No longer is the laboratory a sea of beakers and test tubes. Modern analytical methods involve the use of sophisticated instruments: gas chromatographs, mass spectrometers, and atomic absorption spectrometers. Analyses cost hundreds of dollars per sample. In sampling programs at major sites that involve many monitoring wells, many contaminants, and many sampling rounds, analytical budgets can run into the hundreds of thousands of dollars per year. There are many possible sources of error in these measurements: improper well construction, poor sampling protocols, sample-handling mix-ups, instrument malfunctions in the lab, analytical errors by lab technicians, and even transcription errors as the measured values make their way through the chain of custody from the field to the lab to the computer database to the final report.

Issues of quality control play a huge part in the design of sampling protocols. Most clients continually test the performance of their laboratories by including blind test samples in each batch of samples that they submit for analysis. These include *blanks* (to see if the lab will report zero concentration for a sample free of all contaminants), *duplicates* (to see if the lab will measure the same concentration on two identical samples), and *spikes* (to see if the lab will match the known concentration of a specially spiked sample). Everyone involved in these field studies is wary of false positives (the determination of a contaminant concentration in the lab that is above the regulatory standard, when in fact the true concentration in the field is below), and false negatives (the determination of a contaminant concentration in the lab that is below the regulatory standard, when the true concentration in the field is above). Many studies of the performance of analytical laboratories have concluded that most data sets are rife with false positives and false negatives. Errors are commonplace and incorrect data contaminates every discussion. It is a sorely contentious issue during negotiations between regulatory agencies and PRPs.

As another example from Table 19, consider the interpretation of the extent of a contaminant plume at a site. Imagine a situation like that shown in Figure 11, which is a map view of a shallow sand-and-gravel aquifer in which a contaminated plume is known to exist. The black dots indicate locations where water samples from monitoring wells have indicated the presence of contamination. The open circles indicate locations where sample analysis has come up clean. Figure 11 shows two interpretations of the measured data. The regulatory interpretation assumes that all of the areas not proven to be clean are dirty, while the PRP interpretation assumes that all of the areas not proven to be dirty are clean. The truth undoubtedly lies somewhere in between, but the uncertainty as to exactly where it lies can be cause for considerable conflict during negotiations between regulators and PRPs.

Worse yet is the occurrence of an unexpected hit at some location

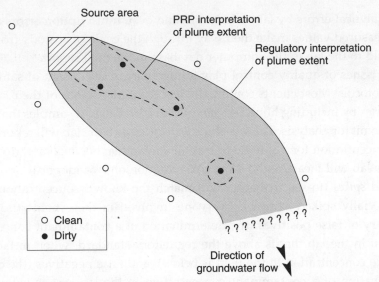

Figure 11.   Plan view of a shallow, contaminated aquifer indicating alternative interpretations of plume extent.

where the existence of the plume has not been suspected or where its presence is highly unlikely. PRPs invariably argue that this is an obvious case of a false positive. Regulatory agencies invariably require costly additional site investigation before they are willing to lay it to rest.

Given the uncertainty that exists in the interpretation of environmental conditions, there is room for multiple hypotheses to come under consideration. One side might argue that the data indicates that there is no offsite migration of contaminants from a site, while the other side might argue that there almost surely is such migration, but that the monitoring network is inadequate to detect it. Not only will the parties disagree over these hypotheses, but they may even disagree over how to deal with the uncertainty that these alternative hypotheses reflect. For example, let me take as my hypothesis that there is no offsite migration. The regulatory agency will want to minimize the possibility of accepting a hypothesis that is false (what statisticians call a Type I Error). In judicial terms, they want to minimize the possibility of letting the guilty party get away scot-free. They will demand further site investigation. The PRP, on the other hand, will want to minimize the possibility of rejecting a hypothesis that is true (a Type II Error). They want to insure that there is no punishment of the innocent. They will argue that further investigation is a form of economic punishment. Even when there is agreement over the level of uncertainty that exists, there may still be conflict over how to deal with it.

The other source of disagreement and conflict in environmental negotiation is the existence of social bias on the part of many of the participants in the environmental game. Sociologists who study interpersonal conflict have identified four different types of social bias, with many subtypes that fall under these four headings.[6] Table 20 lists some of the types of social bias that can lead to breakdowns in environmental negotiations.

A cognitive bias is one that a negotiator may hold without knowing it. His conscious beliefs simply do not reflect the available information. Anyone who has sat through a PTA meeting or an organizational meeting for a Little League baseball team will be familiar with anchoring, where one or more of the participants is so in love with his or her original interpretations and hypotheses that this person fails to take into account the contrary evidence of new information. (Of course, it is best if the participant in question is not oneself.)

A motivational bias is more destructive because it represents a malicious intent to deceive. Management bias, wherein a negotiator's position is biased toward the client's wishes, is particularly common in environmental negotiations.

Some bias may be due to fundamental values. Technical people tend to be utilitarian, pressing for solutions that are somehow societally optimal by maximizing the net value of the costs and benefits of all the individuals in society. Regulatory personnel are often more egalitarian, willing to err on the side of overprotection of those threatened by environmental degradation. Many businesspeople are libertarian in outlook, emphasizing individual rights and wary of costly social programs.

Lastly, there is the corrosive impact of bias due to personality conflict. One sees it in town council meetings on TV. One sees it in the council

Table 20 Examples of social bias that can lead to breakdowns in environmental negotiations.

Cognitive bias:
  Negotiator's conscious beliefs do
  not reflect available information
	Anchoring: insufficient adjustment of
	  initial estimates in light of new
	  information
	Personal bias: tendency to weigh too
	  heavily an event that has personal
	  significance

Motivational bias:
  Negotiator's statements and
  conscious beliefs are inconsistent
	Management bias: interpretations biased
	  toward client's wishes
	Group dynamics bias: the desire to
	  please a dominant leader
	Personal benefit bias: due to personal
	  reward structure
	Conservative bias: err on the safe side

Bias due to values	Utilitarian: maximizes sum of individual
	  costs and benefits
	Egalitarian: desire to protect the least
	  well-off in society
	Libertarian: emphasis on individual
	  rights

Bias due to personality conflict	

meetings at one's condominium. It is no less common in environmental negotiations. It can curtail consensus in a particularly destructive way.

So, with all this discussion in hand, and having had a few years to think about it, I can now give my long-delayed answer to the judge's question. I believe that it is the misuse of technical uncertainty and the festering of social bias that breed disagreement and thwart consensus in environmental negotiations, both in and out of court. If I were still in court I would want a big blowup of Figure 12 in order to illustrate my argument. Suppose, for example, that the question under discussion pertains to the distance that a contaminant plume has migrated away from its source area. We saw in Figure 11 how uncertainty over this issue can

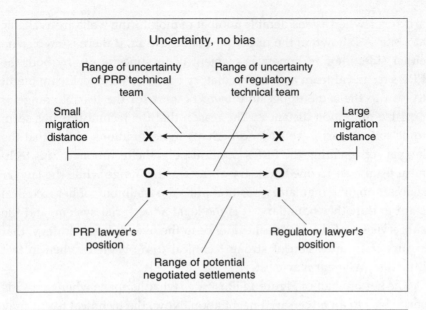

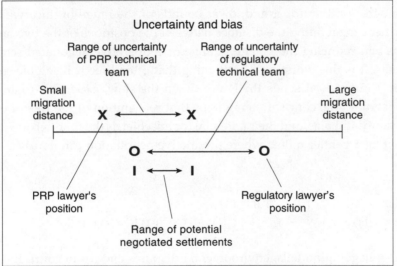

Figure 12. The effect of technical uncertainty and social bias on environmental litigation and negotiation.

arise even when a considerable number of monitoring wells are available at a site. As shown in the upper part of Figure 12, if there is no bias on either side, then an honest assessment of the uncertainty by both the PRP's technical team and the regulatory agency's technical team ought to lead to the same upper and lower bounds for the feasible range of possible migration distances. The reason that the technical teams seem to be so far apart in court (and perhaps in negotiations too) is that the lawyer representing the PRP's position pulls the testimony of his technical team over to one boundary of the feasible range while the lawyer representing the regulatory position pulls the testimony of her technical team to the other boundary. It is the legal adversarial system, and the subservience of the technical evidence to the overall legal strategy, that creates the impression of strong technical disagreement when in fact little disagreement may exist.

The bottom half of Figure 12 illustrates what happens when one adds social bias to an adversarial negotiation. Now, the technical teams may not agree on the upper and lower bounds of the range of uncertainty, further exaggerating the distance between the positions of the two lawyers and reducing the potential range of cooperative negotiated settlements. It is this worst-case positioning that often breeds insoluble conflict. Ultimately it sends the issues down the slow, expensive route of litigation in the courts. It is my hope that recognition of the role of uncertainty and bias, and their potential for mischief, is the first step toward creating a gentler milieu where productive negotiation can flourish.[7]

SEARCHING FOR TRUTH: ENVIRONMENTAL SCIENCE IN THE COURTS

When negotiation fails, environmental disputes end up in court. Regulatory agencies sue PRPs to prove culpability and recover costs. PRPs sue insurance companies to make them honor their policies. One PRP may sue another PRP in order to bring that party to the negotiating table. Environmental groups have been known to sue regulatory agencies to compel them to enforce environmental laws.

Some of these cases are brought to court under the criminal justice system, in which malfeasance must be proven "beyond a reasonable doubt." More often, they are brought to court under the civil justice system, in which the standard of proof is much weaker. A civil case is proven if it is supported by a "preponderance of the evidence" or if it is "more likely than not." It is much easier to convince a judge or jury that one's interpretation is "more likely than not," than it is to convince them that it is true "beyond a reasonable doubt."

High-profile cases are often brought before juries, but most environmental lawsuits are decided by a judge acting alone. Cases are often fought in front of an administrative law judge or, if the case falls under the western water statutes, in front of a court-appointed master.

The outcome of environmental litigation often hangs on the interpretation of technical evidence, and here one finds the courts facing a fundamental conflict between two very different methods of searching for the truth. The expert witnesses hired to present the technical evidence in court anticipate that the methods of science will be used to decide the scientific questions. However, the lawyers are in charge in the legal adversarial milieu, and in this forum presentation and credibility are at least as important as good science.

In their own marketplace, scientific theories gain credence through open discussion and the cumulative buildup of evidence in the published literature. Scientists must convince a large majority of their peers if they want their arguments to be fully accepted. Although not free of conflict, the scientific process is at root a cooperative social venture. The legal milieu is very different. It is adversarial to the core: the truth is reached through structured conflict. Social consensus is not necessary. In a case to be decided by judge alone, there is only one person to convince. Lawyers spend a lot of time and money researching the background, preferences, and biases of any judge they will face, and they then try to spin their case to meet this profile. Scientists, thinking that their evidence is value-free, are likely to be uneasy with this type of legal maneuvering.

Scientists and engineers see their professional relationship with clients quite differently than do lawyers. Engineers expect to provide their client with the technical facts, regardless of whether they provide good news or bad with respect to their client's legal position. They expect to tell the whole story from the witness stand. They may be offended by the careful scripting of their testimony by their client's legal team. Lawyers want to know all the facts, of course, but only so they won't be caught off guard by the opposing counsel. The only facts they will expose in court of their own free will are those that are favorable to their client. In fact, to do otherwise would be unethical. Under the Code of Professional Responsibility of the American Bar Association, "a lawyer should represent a client zealously within the bounds of the law."[8] Scientists and engineers who act as expert witnesses have to remember that "the role of counsel is not to make sure the truth is ascertained but to advance his client's position."[9]

Despite this uneasy alliance, 86 percent of today's civil cases involve expert testimony.[10] The courts increasingly depend on scientific experts. And it is not only in the courts. Expert testimony is also solicited in the course of negotiated settlements. Experts are brought in to support the arguments of one side or the other with respect to such issues as the appropriateness of sites for new waste-management facilities, the need for additional site characterization at new or contaminated sites, the appropriateness of various remedial design alternatives, and the apportionment of costs at sites with multiple responsible parties.

Expert witnesses often find themselves in awkward circumstances. Many legal cases are fought over words that do not have a proper technical definition—whether two events are "connected," for example, or whether a contamination event was "sudden and unexpected."

Environmental scientists and engineers acting as expert witnesses may find themselves walking a thin line with respect to the guidelines for ethical practice of their profession. In the Code of Ethics of the American Society of Civil Engineers, for example, it is stated that engineers "shall not participate in the dissemination of untrue, unfair or exaggerated statements"; that they "shall include all relevant and pertinent information in all reports, statements and testimony"; and that they "shall not accept professional commissions under circumstances in which their professional judgment may be compromised."[11] Unfortunately, exaggeration, selectivity, and compromised judgments are the very stuff of modern legal testimony.

From a lawyer's perspective, the expert witness is simply a "saxophone"—the lawyer calls the tune and the expert plays it.[12] The ideal expert witness is "neat but not dapper, respectable but not pompous, mature but not senile."[13] A former president of the American Bar Association has been quoted as saying that he would go into a lawsuit with an objective, uncommitted, independent expert about as willingly as he would occupy a foxhole with a couple of noncombatant soldiers.[14]

Under these circumstances, where lawyers view scientific impartiality as a character flaw, it is perhaps not surprising that there is an active market for expert witnesses willing to sell their souls. Peter W. Huber, in his book *Galileo's Revenge: Junk Science in the Courtroom*, describes the role of fringe scientists who have sufficient credibility to be qualified as experts and who provide support for positions not accepted by mainstream science.[15] They do so by giving greater weight than is warranted to unpublished experiments that have not undergone the usual rigorous peer review process that accompanies scientific publication. And with the fierce cross-examination that usually accompanies technical testimony, juries often cannot tell the difference between the real scientists and the charlatans. When it suits their needs, lawyers are not above playing on the anti-elitist proclivities of the jury.

The courts have made many attempts to try to separate valid science from speculative opinion.[16] The Frye test, first laid down in 1923, states that scientific testimony must be "sufficiently established to have gained general acceptance in a particular field to which it belongs." Under the U.S. Federal Rules of Evidence introduced in 1975, scientific testimony must be "helpful and reliable" and must "assist in understanding the evidence or to determine a fact." Under this code, judges have the ability to limit the admissibility of evidence if it will "cause confusion or unfair prejudice." In practice, these qualitative admonitions have not proven all that helpful. Other suggestions that have been put forward for improving the quality of technical testimony in court include judges' direct utilization of their own independent experts (an action allowed under current practice but seldom used) and a protocol that would allow judges to demand that lawyers expose all the expert opinions they have solicited, not only the ones that support their case. These suggestions tend to come from the scientific community, who would like to force the courts into their belief system. They are strongly opposed by the legal community, most of whom have a sincere and fervent belief in the efficiency of the adversarial search for truth. It may be cynical to say so, but presumably trial lawyers also see quite clearly that their interests will not be served by a breakdown in the adversarial nature of the current legal framework.

There is a faint silver lining in all of this. In my experience, the courts usually recognize junk science for what it is, and ultimately they seem to reach decisions that would be viewed as technically correct by an objective technical observer. There seems to be a recognition that legal decisions that fly in the face of scientific knowledge will harm both science and the law.[17] It is, however, a costly and time-consuming path to the truth. It is incumbent on all those involved in the environmental game, including those in the legal community, to try to reduce the social costs of pollution by improving the climate for successful negotiation and avoiding the nonproductive morass of litigation.

THE EFFECT OF IMPASSE ON PREVENTIVE ACTION

The public is understandably frustrated with the slow pace of progress in addressing its concerns about environmental degradation. Why, it asks, should it take twelve years from the time a contaminated site is identified under Superfund legislation until a Record of Decision is reached? What produces this incredible inertia?

In the foregoing sections I have tried to identify some of the issues that thwart consensus and delay solutions. I have explored some of the roadblocks to successful negotiation and pointed out the inefficiency of litigative solutions through the courts. These discussions provide a partial explanation, but they are not the whole answer. Unfortunately, delay has become a purposeful strategy on the part of many of the players in the environmental game. There are no good guys and bad guys here. When it suits their needs, all the main players have learned "the fine art of delay."[18]

When it comes to the siting of new waste-management facilities, it is the environmentalists and NIMBY groups that want delay. Back in the early days of the environmental movement, they fought hard to ensure the passage of legislation that mandates a complex and lengthy environmental review process. This process usually requires the preparation of environmental impact statements by the protagonists at one or more stages in the proceedings, and it is almost always designed to allow frequent public participation. Environmentalists argue that strong dependence on formal environmental impact statements protects the environment, and that heavy reliance on public participation is in keeping with our principles of participatory democracy. And so they are. But the process can be misused when it leads to obfuscation for its own sake. A proposed waste-management project should stand or fall on its own merits as part of an overall community waste-management strategy. Once a community's elected representatives have decided that a project should stand, then further attempts to kill it through obstructive delaying tactics are likely to be against the greater environmental good.

When it comes to the cleanup of contaminated sites, the shoe is on the other foot. In this case, it is industry that works for delay. Potentially responsible parties may ignore regulatory requests for information, hire lawyers to provoke procedural delays, delay site characterization activities, overemphasize technical difficulties, and play their political trump cards in the press by threatening bankruptcy and loss of jobs. From the PRP perspective there are two main motives for delay. One is the desire to postpone heavy remedial expenditures to the distant future, and the other is the hope that requirements for site cleanup may soften in the future. Because of the uncertainties in the future regulatory climate, many companies do not record all their known environmental liabilities on their financial statements.[19] If these remedial liabilities are not on the balance sheet, there is little internal incentive for companies to engage in cleanup. It is less costly for the owners of contaminated sites to postpone cleanup through litigation than to initiate remediation.

The result of all this delay is that developers can't get their new facilities under way, and environmentalists can't get polluters to clean up their mess at old facilities. Neither type of delay serves the public interest. I suppose that there are some cases where it might be argued that delay has been beneficial. There have undoubtedly been ill-considered new waste-management facilities that have been scuppered by procedural delay. And there may well be cases where the delay of remedial cleanup saved public money by avoiding useless expenditures on sites that offered no environmental risk. More often, however, the delay of new waste-management facilities simply encourages inappropriate or illegal waste disposal elsewhere; and delay in containment of contaminated sites simply leads to further offsite migration and greater threats to drinking-water supplies.

More important, delays in remedial action generally also delay preventive action. Preventive activities such as the replacement of leaky underground tanks, the refurbishing of old industrial facilities, and the improvement of protocols for the response to accidental chemical spills tend to get caught in any overall industrial strategy of delay. Regardless of how one might feel about the delay of remedial action, there is no doubt that the delay of preventive action is very much against the public interest. Regardless of how regulatory agencies may react to industrial delaying tactics over remediation of contaminated sites, it is imperative that the pace of improvement in preventive action not be compromised.

ETHICAL CONUNDRUMS

Ethical dilemmas lurk in the wings for all of the players in the environmental game. I noted earlier the differences between technical ethics and legal ethics in the representation of client interests. How should technical advisors and expert witnesses cope with legal recommendations that are legally ethical but may not be ethical in a technical sense? Withholding or suppressing information from the opposition through legal privilege, for example, may be a proper and acceptable legal maneuver, but it may cause ethical concerns to a scientist or engineer. Is it ethical for a geologist to accept a legal recommendation to stop a site drilling program when more data would clarify the technical issues, but where bad news might harm the client's interests? Is it ethical for an engineer to take part in legal proceedings in support of a client's interests if she does not believe that a favorable decision would be in the public interest?

Environmental scientists and engineers also face ethical concerns because of the heavy layer of regulation that now blankets all environmental issues. The first fundamental canon in the Code of Ethics of the American Society of Civil Engineers states that engineers "shall hold paramount the safety, health, and welfare of the public in the performance of their professional duties."[20] In the absence of regulations, the design engineer would presumably prepare designs for a waste-management facility that are in keeping with his interpretation of the Code of Ethics. However, with a detailed regulatory system in place, most design engineers will probably feel that they have satisfied their ethical obligations if they meet the regulatory requirements. Certainly, this seems to be the prevailing view in the nuclear-waste and hazardous-waste industries. It raises the question as to how an engineer should act if he or she believes that the regulations are inadequate. One can only imagine how the client would likely react if the design engineer were to recommend spending large additional sums of money to exceed the regulatory design standards just for peace of mind. The point is that an engineering ethic cannot be viewed as morally absolute: it is a function of the regulatory climate.

There are many types of behavior by technical advisors that are clearly unethical: bending interpretations to meet a client's wishes; bending interpretations to meet personal, political, or social beliefs; failing to report serious technical reservations about site interpretations or proposed remedial designs; using one's personal credibility to bolster a weak technical position; and taking advantage of a weak technical adversary. One recent editorial on this topic argues that overzealous advocacy for a client's position is the most common ethical transgression on the part of engineering consultants, and that the recent decline in the environmental market with its increased competition for consulting work has placed increased pressures on technical consultants to please their clients.[21] In the results of a recent questionnaire published in an engineering news-letter, almost a quarter of those engineers surveyed answered the question "Have you ever been subjected to pressure to professionally certify findings that you did not agree with?" in the affirmative.[22]

Owner-operators of waste-management sites are open to many ethical temptations. If not morally constrained, it can be to a firm's economic advantage to violate pollution control laws. Under the current funding levels in the regulatory community, the probability that an illegal release will be detected by the regulators may be relatively low; and even if detected, there may be inadequate follow-through on enforcement. The violation of pollution standards under lax enforcement is clearly unethical. Some managers will defend themselves on the grounds that the regulations are unfair, but this is not a persuasive argument. Unfair regulations should be fought politically or procedurally, not through lack of compliance.

Regulatory agencies are not free from unethical behavior. They deal with a large number of contamination incidents and they encounter a wide spectrum of cooperation, or lack thereof, from the owner-operators in the negotiations leading to remedial action. In general, regulatory agencies have not been willing to distinguish between good and bad corporate citizens in their regulatory protocols. They resist identifying cooperative firms to the public for fear of being accused of being in bed with the polluters. The result is that potentially harmonious and efficient cleanup procedures are turned into acrimonious conflicts for political reasons. If the firms perceive that there is no advantage to cooperation, even the good corporate citizens are unlikely to take a positive stance in future dealings with regulatory agencies. Government dishonesty as to the level of cooperation given by polluting companies is unethical, and it has a social cost.

Lastly, there are the special interest groups. They too are not immune to unethical behavior. There can be a level and style of advocacy on the part of environmental groups that is unethical. If the true aims of the group are different from the stated ones, if facts that are known to be false are presented as true, in short, if the end justifies the means, then such advocacy is unethical.

One would like to think that unethical behavior, regardless of the source, receives its just rewards. In the long run I suspect that this is so, but in the short run unethical behavior has great potential to play havoc with our system of social decision-making. I have no solutions to suggest other than to add my voice to the growing clamor for a return to a higher moral standard in everyday business affairs. The decline in ethical standards is affecting society on a much broader front than is commonly recognized.

ENVIRONMENTAL CRIME

There is a line, and once one steps across it, unethical behavior becomes criminal behavior. Like all criminals, environmental criminals come in many shades: from petty criminals just barely over the line, to international organized crime preying on society.

The lowest level of environmental crime is illegal dumping of waste by individuals. It is one of those slightly antisocial actions that doesn't seem very serious when one person does it once (especially if the person is oneself). However, when a lot of people do it a lot of times, it becomes a social problem. A survey in Tucson, Arizona, found seventeen hundred small illegal dumps in the vicinity of the city.[23] Apparently the temptation to avoid the tipping fees at licensed landfills is just too great for many people, especially when the activity is viewed as only marginally illegal and the probability of apprehension is slight. The closure of landfills is also a contributing factor. Studies have shown that when a local landfill closes, many new illegal dumps are spawned nearby.

Small firms that produce limited quantities of hazardous waste are also prone to temptation. As the number of licensed disposal facilities has gone down, and as the tipping fees at the facilities that remain have gone up, there has been a documented increase in illegal dumping of industrial hazardous waste across the nation. In Illinois, for example, in the mid-1980s, there were twenty-two approved chemical landfills that received approximately 2 million tons of waste per year. The problem is that reliable estimates of the total waste generated in Illinois run many times higher than this, and no one really knows where the rest of it went.[24]

Michael Brown, in his influential book *Laying Waste: The Poisoning of America by Toxic Chemicals*, documents a variety of illegal activities associated with waste management.[25] They range from small-scale "midnight haulers" to large-scale infiltration of the industry by organized crime. The potential for illegal profit is immense. Because the cost of legally disposing of a drum of chemical waste is now so high ($100 per drum, or more), midnight haulers can easily undercut the going price and then simply dump the waste in a back-road ditch at essentially no cost. There are many horror stories on record of hazardous-waste tanker trucks cruising the nation's turnpikes in the dark of night with their valves open.[26] The organized-crime families that control this illegal business contract the dirty work out to small-time truckers, who change their company names every time the law gets close, painting and repainting their trucks with alacrity and eluding enforcement through the loopholes of corporate identity. Most midnight haulers are never caught, and those that do fall into the hands of the law are seldom given jail terms or charged fines anywhere near large enough to cover the costs of cleaning up the mess that they have created.

There is a strong argument to be made that it is in the best interests of society to make the hazardous-waste-management business profitable.[27] If it is not, many companies capable of providing the technical skills needed for hazardous-waste disposal will avoid this opportunity because of its high visibility and the associated notoriety in the event of an accident. If reputable companies avoid the field, the demand will be filled by disreputable companies. If enforcement of environmental statutes is uncertain due to underfunding, then illegal suppliers of waste-management services will thrive.

One of the most disturbing developments in recent years has been the growth in international trafficking in hazardous waste.[28] As the developed nations like Canada, the United States, and the countries of western Europe develop tighter and tighter regulations on the disposal of hazardous waste, there is a temptation for international companies to ship their waste across international borders to countries in Latin America and eastern Europe where waste disposal takes place under more lenient rules.

There may also be traffic in the other direction. Chemicals that have been banned in the developed countries are often still available in the third world. In one recent case, the U.S. government filed charges against twelve people for smuggling chlorofluorocarbons (CFCs) from Mexico into the United States.[29] These chemicals, the most common of which is known as Freon, are refrigerants for automobile air conditioners, but they have been banned in the United States as a threat to the ozone layer. Smugglers buy the CFCs for $4 a kilo in Mexico and sell them for $25 to $40 a kilo on the American black market, where they are still in demand by owners of U.S. cars built before 1994.

The Environmental Protection Agency tries valiantly to enforce its statutes, but neither the local offices nor the National Enforcement Investigation Center in Colorado is able to meet all of the EPA's nationwide enforcement responsibilities for RCRA, the Superfund, and other environmental laws, both national and international. Between 1983 and 1995, the EPA and the Department of Justice prosecuted 1,481 criminal cases, obtaining 1,074 pleas and convictions, $300 million in criminal fines, and a total of 561 person-years of prison time.[30] This seems like a reasonable record until one looks at the details. The longest sentence ever received for an environmental crime is twenty-seven months, and it went to a self-employed truck mechanic for placing topsoil in a wetland. Many of the prosecutions are for technical violations of the laws by otherwise reputable companies, rather than for serious cases of illegal dumping by midnight haulers and organized crime. There is a tendency to enforce and prosecute those cases that appear winnable at the expense of those more difficult cases that represent the greatest threat to the environment.

The challenge to the regulatory agencies is great. They must put in place a set of regulations and an enforcement procedure that protects the health and safety of the public and discourages the criminal element, yet allows for a healthy return on investment by reputable businesses. If the public does not support a sufficient level of funding for the agencies, the agencies will be forced to choose between a system of slack enforcement of stringent regulations or strong enforcement of weak regulations. The first will lead to environmental pollution from illegal sources; the second will lead to pollution from poorly designed facilities.

THE BOTTOM LINE

• The environmental game involves unavoidable adversarial conflict between regulatory agencies and industrial corporations. It is in the societal interest that the two sides receive equally strong technical and legal advice. To this end, it is incumbent on regulatory agencies to keep their salary structures competitive with industry in order to stem the current drain of talented technical and legal personnel from government service into the private sector.

• Environmental decisions that are unilaterally handed down by regulatory agencies without negotiation and against the wishes of the regulated community are seldom successfully implemented. The industrial backlash usually leads to technical and legal gridlock.

• Judicial decisions handed down in a court of law as a result of litigation between the parties are usually implementable, but the judicial route is inefficient, costly, and time-consuming. It is incumbent on all parties to an environmental conflict, including those in the legal community, to try to reduce the current dependence on litigated solutions.

• A negotiated settlement between the parties is the most desirable path to an environmental decision. The most common roadblocks to consensus involve disagreements over the importance of site uncertainties and the festering of long-held institutional biases.

• Environmental scientists and engineers acting as expert witnesses on behalf of interested parties in hearings and court cases often find themselves facing ethical dilemmas with respect to the nature of their involvement and the use of their technical findings. The quality of technical testimony in such cases would probably be improved if judges relied more on their own independent experts.

• The art of delay has become a purposeful strategy on the part of many of the players in the environmental game. It is imperative that such delaying tactics not be allowed to shut down the much-needed siting of new waste-management facilities, nor to slow the pace of preventive remedial action at industrial sites.

- It is in the best interests of society that the hazardous-waste-management business be profitable. If it is not, reputable companies will avoid the field, and the demand will be filled by disreputable companies. It is equally important that regulatory agencies be funded at a sufficient level to allow them to firmly enforce the laws against illegal suppliers of waste-management services.

- There is a need for a high moral standard on the part of all the parties to environmental disputes in their everyday business dealings with one another. The decline in business morality is a serious national concern, and there is evidence of this decline in the environmental sector, just as in the more traditional sectors of the business community.

8 Solutions

In the past thirty years we have come full circle. We have seen the environmental pendulum swing across the full arc of potential environmental policies: from underkill to overkill, from conditions of environmental degradation and the attendant threat to human health, to a situation where overconservative risk aversion has led to the waste of public monies in the service of inappropriate regulation.

The sweep of the pendulum has polarized the environmental perspectives. On one end of the arc, we have the Greenpeace perspective, which paints corporate America as an indifferent band of careless polluters; at the other end, we have the perspective of the new right, which views the environmental movement as some kind of anti-free-enterprise plot.

I hope that our quest for the truth will lead all of us to reject both of these extreme positions. We need a more pragmatic and workable approach to environmental protection, one that meets societal demands for the reduction of health risk, but recognizes the unavoidability of hazardous waste and our need to dispose of it; one that recognizes the need to protect the environment from unacceptable degradation but at the same time maintain the economic health of the nation.

As we come to the turn of the century, there is reason for optimism. Corporations are buying into the environmental ethic. Regulatory agencies are softening their position. There is potential for a more cooperative milieu among the parties, based on a balanced and participatory approach to negotiation, and less reliance on legal adversarial conflict.

In this final chapter we review the bad news and the good news, and we look at some steps that might take us in the right direction toward more effective environmental policies.

THE BAD NEWS

- There is a suite of chemicals composed primarily of chlorinated organics and metals known to be toxic and/or carcinogenic when experienced in acute doses by human beings. These chemicals appear in the waste streams of many industrial processes that produce the consumer goods that drive our material way of life.

- Hazardous industrial waste containing toxic organic chemicals is generated at a rate of 250 million tons per year in the United States. The rates of generation are more likely to increase than decrease in the future.

- Contaminant releases to the environment arise from improper waste disposal practices and from accidental spills and leaks during the operation of industrial plants. Even small releases can have a large environmental impact.

- Across the country there are tens of thousands of sites contaminated with toxic chemicals. These sites are a legacy of inappropriate waste disposal practices in the early years of the chemical revolution.

- Current industrial practices will reduce but not eliminate future chemical releases into the environment. Small releases are probably unavoidable in the course of normal industrial operations.

- Any realistic future waste-management strategy for the nation must include continued reliance on land-based disposal as one component in the mix of waste-disposal technologies.

- Modern landfills with their improved design specifications are much less likely to leak over the short term than poorly designed older landfills. However, even the most well-constructed landfill has a finite life expectancy after which it can be expected to fail. Current design practice delays, attenuates, and possibly reduces contaminant releases to the environment, but it does not prevent them forever.

- Recycling is not a panacea. Even under the most optimistic scenarios, recycling can handle only a small percentage of the total waste load generated. It will not negate the need for the siting of new landfills for industrial and municipal waste.

- The inability of our current political framework to provide proper siting of new waste-management facilities encourages unacceptable practices that expose the public to greater health risks than would accrue from properly sited facilities.

- There are no current or emerging technologies that can achieve the necessary recovery rates in the removal of contamination from contaminated sites. Source-area restoration is neither technically nor economically feasible, nor is it likely to become so in the foreseeable future.

- Site containment without source removal requires a commitment on the part of both industry and regulatory agencies to maintain control over contaminated sites in perpetuity. It remains to be seen whether these organizations have the will to fund and administer environmental programs that have no end.

- There are so many environmental regulations now in place, and so many different agencies administering them, that full compliance with all municipal, state, and federal laws may well be impossible. The lack of integration across these regulatory programs often leads to inconsistent enforcement and unintended environmental consequences.

- There are social costs associated with both underkill and overkill in the enforcement of policies designed to provide environmental protection. The social costs of underkill are environmental degradation and unacceptable impacts on human health. The social costs of over-kill include the diversion of resources from areas of greater need.

• Objective assessments of a wide suite of risk-reducing regulations in-dicate that many environmental regulations aimed at control of toxic chemicals are less effective than regulations that provide more direct impact on health and safety.

THE GOOD NEWS

• In general, public health is improving, not deteriorating. Life expec-tancy continues to increase, and the quality of life in later years con-tinues to improve.

• The risk of acute exposure to toxic chemicals (including pesticides, PCBs, lead, and dioxins) has been much reduced over the years.

• While there is still a degree of uncertainty as to the level of risk asso-ciated with long-term, low-dose, chronic exposures to environmental chemicals, there are very few documented cases of health impacts from such exposures. If there has been any significant increase in the incidence of cancer or other serious diseases due to environmental degradation, the effect has been very small. The impact of toxic chemicals on human health is orders of magnitude less than the im-pact of other cultural activities, such as smoking.

• Experts in societal risk assessment do not perceive the risks associ-ated with environmental chemicals and contaminated sites to be very high relative to other risks. They do not regard chemical haz-ardous waste as a major long-term public health threat.

• If new waste management facilities are sited in favorable hydrogeo-logical settings, then it is very unlikely that contamination from such facilities will threaten water-supply aquifers.

• The primary exposure path leading to potentially harmful human health impact due to environmental contamination occurs through the ingestion of contaminated drinking water from groundwater aquifers that are impacted by contaminated sites. Fortunately, only a small percentage of historically contaminated sites actually threaten public drinking-water supplies. Many contaminated sites are fortui-tously located in favorable hydrogeological settings and thus pose very little risk to public health.

- There are many contaminated sites where the natural biodegradation of petroleum hydrocarbon contaminants has led to sufficient attenuation of plume-migration rates to eliminate the threat of aquifer contamination.

- At those historical sites where favorable circumstances are not present, and in the absence of suitable restoration technologies, there are nevertheless several commercially available technologies that represent viable options for source-area containment. At most sites it is now possible to attain hydraulic control by means of pump-and-treat systems, physical control by means of cutoff walls, chemical control through the use of reactive barriers, or biological control through engineered bioremediation.

SOME STEPS IN THE RIGHT DIRECTION

The most important steps in the right direction must come from the legislators who codify environmental policy into legislation and set up the regulatory framework for its enforcement.

- Environmental policy should emphasize prevention of future contamination rather than remediation of historical contamination. Prevention is at least an order of magnitude more cost-effective than remediation. The current overemphasis on remedial action has unrecognized social costs, not the least of which is the diversion of resources from other environmental programs that address issues of greater concern, including air pollution, ozone depletion, and global warming.

- An environmental policy that encourages proper technical siting of waste-management facilities represents the single most important step that could be taken to protect the environment from contamination.

- Environmental policy should stress aquifer protection and watershed control rather than individual site cleanup.

- Recycling is an important and valuable component in the mix of waste-management strategies needed to keep our waste problems under control. There is still considerable scope for the enhancement of both municipal and industrial recycling activities.

- There remains a need for strong contaminated-sites regulation. Current contaminated-sites regulation has created conditions of over-regulation that are not in the public interest. However, current thrusts toward deregulation have become too ideological. What is needed is not abandonment of the legislation but fine-tuning to avoid remedial overkill.

- The maximum contaminant levels (MCLs) that have been established for toxic chemicals may be appropriate for deciding on the potability of public water supplies, but they are too conservative to act as appropriate compliance targets for cleanup at contaminated industrial sites that do not threaten drinking-water sources. Their use at such sites has led to unacceptable waste of public and private monies.

- The specific needs for regulatory rationalization of contaminated-sites legislation include: (1) the need to reevaluate the Priority Pollutants List with an eye to removing some of the more benign toxicants from it, (2) the need to relax the MCLs for many chemicals, (3) the need to replace MCL-driven cleanups at contaminated sites with risk-based decision processes, (4) the need to bring acceptable-risk levels in environmental matters into balance with the risk levels that are accepted in other walks of life, and (5) the need to move away from source-area restoration technologies toward containment technologies.

- Prevention of environmental degradation would be more effective if it were carried out in a cooperative regulatory framework using a softer and fairer doctrine of liability. The lack of moral justice in the retroactive and joint-and-several liability provisions in the Superfund legislation has provoked resistance and obstruction on the part of the potentially responsible parties at contaminated sites. The detrimental effects of the resulting legal gridlock outweigh the value of any added cost recovery that can be achieved through the application of these liability doctrines.

- Regulatory policies must allow for a healthy return on investment by reputable waste-management companies so that disreputable companies are not attracted into the business. It is equally important that regulatory agencies be funded at a sufficient level to allow them to firmly enforce the laws against illegal suppliers of waste-management services.

- Legislators from all jurisdictions must recognize the need for policy integration to avoid overlap, duplication, and inefficiency.

- Societal cost-benefit analysis should be used to prioritize environmental laws and to compare the value of environmental legislation relative to other risk-reducing and health-enhancing legislation.

In addition to these direct legislative recommendations, there are also steps that could be taken by regulatory agencies to improve the effectiveness of the programs set up to implement environmental legislation.

- Regulatory agencies should try to develop an enforcement milieu that encourages cooperation and compromise with industrial corporations rather than adversarial conflict. Society would be better served by a framework that emphasizes negotiated settlements rather than judicial settlements that arise from costly, time-consuming litigation.
- The prioritization of contaminated sites for remedial attention should be based on health risk. Agencies should resist politically driven priority setting.
- Remedial action at large contaminated sites that threaten drinking-water supplies should be based on containment rather than restoration. In most cases, restoration is neither technically nor economically feasible. It must be recognized that most source areas will remain toxic in perpetuity, and this creates the need for long-term monitoring and enforcement.
- Remedial decisions should be based on a site-specific assessment of health risk rather than on blind adherence to compliance standards. However, current protocols that use unrealistic receptor scenarios in a worst-case risk analysis are not appropriate. They lead to a significant overestimation of the health risks at contaminated sites and over-expenditure of scarce environmental funding that could be better spent elsewhere.
- Remedial decisions at contaminated sites should take future land use into account. It is not economically or technically feasible to return heavily contaminated industrial sites to pristine conditions.
- It is incumbent on regulatory agencies to keep their salary structures competitive with industry in order to stem the current drain of talented technical and legal personnel from government service into the private sector.

There are also steps that can be taken by many of the other players in the environmental game.

- The technical community should make an effort to raise the scientific awareness of the public by providing the media with facts about environmental problems and specific contamination incidents. They should be forthright about the level of technical uncertainty that underlies their recommendations, and the expected longevity of engineered solutions.

- The legal community should provide greater support to the search for negotiated settlements and try to reduce the current dependence on inefficient litigated solutions.

- The media should make a greater effort to learn the facts about environmental controversies. They should abandon good-guy/bad-guy stereotypes and stop providing a forum for maverick scientists under the guise of balance. It may not make as good a story, but the solutions to most technical problems lie with mainstream science and engineering.

Environmentalists have a special role to play in this new era. They deserve the credit for bringing the issues of environmental degradation into the public eye. Now their help is needed in implementing the solutions. It is a time for the environmental movement to move toward a modus operandi of cooperation and compromise rather than confrontation.

- Environmentalists should recognize the public consensus that both environmental health and economic health are important and compatible.

- Environmentalists should help develop and support regional waste-management strategies. They should recognize that environmental activists who oppose all new waste-management facilities are taking action that promotes rather than curtails environmental degradation.

- Environmentalists should be more selective in distinguishing between cases that involve pure NIMBY protest and cases that involve a true environmental threat. They should not allow their support to be misused by NIMBY protesters who try to ride on environmental coattails.

- Environmentalists should be willing to differentiate between good and bad corporate citizens and to inform the press and public about proactive and cooperative companies as well as those that fail to cooperate in environmental remediation.

- There should be continued support and encouragement for recycling, especially in the industrial sector, but its value should be presented to the public as that of a useful component in an overall waste-management strategy, not a self-sufficient panacea.

- Environmentalists should try to lead the public to take greater interest in higher-risk global issues like ozone depletion and global warming, rather than pandering to the public's fears about marginal local risks.

Finally, we come to industry. Here are the parties responsible for most environmental contamination. To a large degree, the question of environmental recovery is in their hands. No matter how strong the environmental activism, nor how tenacious the enforcement of environmental regulations, success is unlikely to be achieved without the cooperation of corporate America.

- Irrespective of the level of regulatory pressure, it is in the best interests of corporations to independently and proactively assess the level of historical contamination at their industrial plants and take the necessary steps to get it under control so that it does not impact surface-water bodies or drinking-water aquifers.

- Companies should upgrade all plant facilities that have the potential to lead to environmental contamination, in particular, underground storage tanks, leaky pipelines, and outdated waste-management facilities.

- It is incumbent on companies to establish effective chemical-spill-prevention and spill-response programs to insure that future incidents do not lead to the unacceptable levels of contamination created by historical carelessness.

- Corporate officers must vigorously defend their environmental programs against the bottom-line demands of shareholders and mutual-fund managers, especially in hard economic times.

- Lastly, corporations must abandon the disruptive, adversarial style of response that has characterized their reaction to regulatory pressure in the past, and enter a new era of cooperation geared to the development of mutually acceptable negotiated settlements.

Sources

CHAPTER 1. THE POLARIZATION
OF THE ENVIRONMENT

1. Harold C. Barnett, *Toxic Debts and the Superfund Dilemma* (Chapel Hill: University of North Carolina Press, 1994), 14.

2. H. W. Lewis, *Technological Risk* (New York: W. W. Norton and Company, 1990), 138.

3. William Rathje and Cullen Murphy, *Rubbish! The Archeology of Garbage* (New York: HarperCollins, 1992), 41.

4. Rachel Carson, *Silent Spring* (Boston: Houghton Mifflin, 1962), 8.

5. Michael D. LaGrega, Phillip L. Buckingham, and Jeffrey C. Evans, *Hazardous Waste Management* (New York: McGraw-Hill, 1994), 5.

6. Ibid.

7. Carson, *Silent Spring,* 43; Leonard F. Konikow and Douglas W. Thompson, "Groundwater Contamination and Aquifer Reclamation at the Rocky Mountain

Arsenal, Colorado," in *Groundwater Contamination* (Washington, D.C.: National Academy Press, 1984), 93–103.

8.   Michael H. Brown, *Laying Waste: The Poisoning of America by Toxic Chemicals* (New York: Pantheon Books, 1979), 173–80.

9.   LaGrega et al., *Hazardous Waste Management*, 7.

10.   James F. Pankow and John A. Cherry, *Dense Chlorinated Solvents and Other DNAPLs in Groundwater: History, Behavior, and Remediation* (Waterloo, Ont.: Waterloo Press, 1996); Robert H. Harris, "Health Risks of Contaminated Groundwater: Real or Imaginary," *GSA Today* 3 (1993): 181–83; Jonathan Harr, *A Civil Action* (New York: Random House, 1995).

11.   John A. Hird, *Superfund: The Political Economy of Environmental Risk* (Johns Hopkins University Press, 1994); Brown, *Laying Waste;* Pierre Berton, *Niagara: A History of the Falls* (Toronto: McClelland and Stewart, 1992); Daniel Mazmanian and David Morell, *Beyond Superfailure: America's Toxics Policy for the 1990s* (Boulder, Colo.: Westview Press, 1992).

12.   Marc Mowrey and Tim Redmond, *Not in Our Backyard: The People and Events That Shaped America's Modern Environmental Movement* (New York: William Morrow and Company, 1993), 39–43.

13.   Ron Arnold, *Ecology Wars: Environmentalism as If People Mattered* (Bellevue, Wash.: Free Enterprise Press, 1993), 29–36; Robert Paehlke, "Environmentalism: Motherhood, Revolution, or Just Plain Politics," *Alternatives* 13 (1985): 29–33.

14.   Barnett, *Toxic Debts*, 17.

15.   LaGrega et al., *Hazardous Waste Management*, 16.

16.   Barnett, *Toxic Debts*, 27.

17.   Ibid., 24.

18.   Mazmanian and Morell, *Beyond Superfailure*, 160–65.

19.   Barnett, *Toxic Debts*, 28.

20.   Harr, *Civil Action*, 208.

21.   LaGrega et al., *Hazardous Waste Management;* Barnett, *Toxic Debts;* U.S. Office of Technology Assessment, *Protecting the Nation's Groundwater from Contamination*, 2 vols. (Washington, D.C.: U.S. Government Printing Office, 1984).

22.   Hird, *Superfund;* LaGrega et al., *Hazardous Waste Management;* Milton E. Russell, William Colglazier, and Mary R. English, *Hazardous Waste Remediation: The Task Ahead* (Knoxville: University of Tennessee at Knoxville, Waste Management Research and Education Institute, 1991).

23.   "Referendums and Other Elections," *USA Today*, November 6, 1996.

24.   Sean Fine, "Canada on Environmental Hotseat," *Toronto Globe and Mail*, July 25, 1997.

25.   Alexander Volokh and Roger Marzulla, *Environmental Enforcement: In Search of Both Effectiveness and Fairness*, Policy Study No. 210 (Los Angeles: Reason Foundation, 1996).

26. Paul R. Ehrlich and Anne H. Ehrlich, *Betrayal of Science and Reason: How Anti-Environmental Rhetoric Threatens Our Future* (Washington, D.C.: Island Press, 1996).

27. Union of Concerned Scientists, *Warning to Humanity* (Cambridge, Mass.: Union of Concerned Scientists, April, 1997).

28. Robert D. Kaplan, *The Ends of the Earth: A Journey to the Frontiers of Anarchy* (New York: Vintage Books, 1996).

29. Lewis, *Technological Risk;* Leonard A. Sagan, *The Health of Nations* (New York: Basic Books, 1987), 4–5; Jay H. Lehr, "Toxicological Risk Assessment Distortions: Parts I, II, and III," *Ground Water* 28 (1990): 2–8, 170–75, 330–40.

30. Sagan, *Health,* 17.

31. Lewis, *Technological Risk,* 5.

32. Sagan, *Health,* 28–41, 186.

33. Lewis, *Technological Risk.*

34. Lehr, "Toxicological Risk," 8.

35. Richard Doll and Richard Peto, *The Causes of Cancer* (New York: Oxford University Press, 1981).

36. Marvin A. Schneiderman, "The Uncertain Risks We Run: Hazardous Materials," in *Societal Risk Assessment: How Safe Is Safe Enough?* ed. Richard C. Schwing and Walter A. Albers Jr. (New York: Plenum Press, 1980), 19–37.

37. Doll and Peto, *Causes of Cancer.*

38. K. S. Shrader-Frechette, *Risk and Rationality: Philosophical Foundations for Populist Reforms* (Berkeley and Los Angeles: University of California Press, 1991).

39. Lehr, "Toxicological Risk."

40. "It's Time to Assess Environmental Policy," *EOS, Transactions American Geophysical Union* 77 (April 30, 1996): 173.

41. William R. Freudenburg, "Strange Chemistry: Environmental Risk Conflicts in a World of Science, Values, and Blind Spots," in *Handbook for Environmental Risk Decision Making: Values, Perceptions, and Ethics,* ed. C. Richard Cothern (Boca Raton: CRC Press, 1996), 11–21.

42. Bruce Yandle, *The Political Limits of Environmental Regulation* (Westport, Conn.: Quorum Books, 1989).

43. W. Spence, R. B. Herrmann, A. C. Johnston, and G. Reagor, "Responses to Iben Browning's Prediction of a 1990 New Madrid, Missouri, Earthquake," U.S. Geological Survey, Circular 1083 (Washington, D.C.: U.S. Government Printing Office, 1993).

44. Lehr, "Toxicological Risk."

45. Harr, *Civil Action.*

46. Lehr, "Toxicological Risk."

47. "Nuclear Explosions in a Geologic Repository? Peer Review Meets Politics

and the Press," *EOS, Transactions American Geophysical Union* 76 (June 20, 1995): 252.

48.   Eldridge M. Moores, "Geology and Culture: A Call for Action," *GSA Today* 7 (January 1997).

49.   Cathy Hainer, "At Peace with Death," *USA Today,* August 11, 1997.

50.   Robert Uhlig, "Aussie Creationist Faces Court Fight over Noah's Ark Claim," *Vancouver Sun,* December 24, 1996.

51.   John Allen Paulos, *Innumeracy: Mathematical Illiteracy and Its Consequences* (New York: Hill and Wang, 1988).

52.   William Back, Edward R. Landa, and Lisa Meeks, "Bottled Water, Spas, and the Early Years of Water Chemistry," *Ground Water* 33 (1995): 605–14.

53.   J. R. Studlick and R. C. Bain, "Bottled Waters: Expensive Ground Water," *Ground Water* 18 (1980): 340–45.

54.   James Flynn, Roger Kasperson, Howard Kunreuther, and Paul Slovic, "Time to Rethink Nuclear Waste Storage," *Issues in Science and Technology* (summer 1992): 42–48.

55.   S. Hilgartner, R. C. Bell, and R. O'Connor, *Nukespeak: The Selling of Nuclear Technology in America* (San Francisco: Sierra Club Books, 1982).

56.   Flynn et al., "Time."

57.   "Public Knows the Value of Science, but Not the Meaning," *EOS, Transactions American Geophysical Union* 77 (August 27, 1996): 339.

58.   Susan Keith, "Science Facts versus Perception in the Public Decision-Making Process," *Ground Water* 24 (1986): 298–301.

59.   Mazmanian and Morell, *Beyond Superfailure,* 184.

60.   "Environmental Industry Hits $180 Billion in Revenues," *Ground Water Monitoring Review* 16 (fall 1996): 4.

61.   LaGrega et al., *Hazardous Waste Management;* Hird, *Superfund.*

62.   "Environmental Industry Hits $180 Billion in Revenues," *Ground Water Monitoring Review* 16 (fall 1996): 4.

63.   David Suzuki, *The Sacred Balance: Rediscovering Our Place in Nature* (Vancouver: Douglas and McIntyre, 1997), 209.

64.   M. E. Pate-Cornell, "Discounting in Risk Analysis: Capital vs Human Safety," in *Risk, Structural Engineering, and Human Error,* ed. M. Grigoriu (Waterloo, Ont.: University of Waterloo Press, 1984), 17–32.

65.   Bayard L. Catron, Lawrence G. Boyer, Jennifer Grund, and John Hartung, "The Problem of Intergenerational Equity: Balancing Risks, Costs, and Benefits Fairly across Generations," in *Handbook for Environmental Risk Decision Making: Values, Perceptions, and Ethics,* ed. C. Richard Cothern (Boca Raton: CRC Press, 1996), 131–48.

66.   Ibid.; R. R. Howarth, "Environmental Risks and Future Generations: Cri-

teria for Public Policy," in *Clean Water and the American Economy*, EPA Report No. 800-R-93-001b, vol. 2 (Washington, D.C.: U.S. Government Printing Office, 1993).

67.   K. Mather, *The Permissive Universe* (Albuquerque: University of New Mexico Press, 1986).

CHAPTER 2.   BLENDERS AND BUICKS:
THE ENVIRONMENTAL CONSEQUENCES
OF OUR ENGINEERED WAY OF LIFE

1.   G. E. Dieter, *Engineering Design: A Materials and Processing Approach* (New York: McGraw-Hill, 1983), 20.

2.   LaGrega et al., *Hazardous Waste Management*, 376–85.

3.   R. R. Affleck, Donald R. Manolescu, and Thomas W. K. Lee, "Closing the Loop: Toward Zero Effluent in Pulp and Paper," *B.C. Professional Engineer* (December 1996): 8–11.

4.   Ibid.

5.   Ford Foundation, *Nuclear Power: Issues and Choices* (Cambridge, Mass.: Ballinger Publishing, 1977), 399–405.

6.   Ibid.; R. C. Schwing, "Trade-Offs," in *Societal Risk Assessment: How Safe Is Safe Enough?* ed. Richard C. Schwing and Walter A. Albers Jr. (New York: Plenum Press, 1980), 129–41.

7.   Zhores Medvedev, *The Legacy of Chernobyl* (New York: W. W. Norton and Company, 1990), 129.

8.   Ibid.

9.   Mazmanian and Morell, *Beyond Superfailure;* LaGrega et al., *Hazardous Waste Management;* Barnett, *Toxic Debts;* Rathje and Murphy, *Rubbish!*

10.   Barnett, *Toxic Debts,* 19.

11.   Rathje and Murphy, *Rubbish!* 49.

12.   Brown, *Laying Waste,* 272.

13.   Rathje and Murphy, *Rubbish!* 50.

14.   Oakhill Environmental, *A Comparison of How Nuclear and Non-nuclear Wastes Are Managed and Disposed* (prepared for the Canadian Federal Panel for the Environmental Assessment of the Nuclear Fuel Waste Management and Disposal Concept, October, 1996).

15.   Rathje and Murphy, *Rubbish!* 181.

16.   G. Fred Lee and R. Anne Jones, "Landfills and Groundwater Quality," *Groundwater* 29 (1991): 482–86.

17.   G. B. Baecher, M. E. Pate, and R. de Neufville, "Risk of Dam Failure in Benefit-Cost Analysis," *Water Resources Research* 16 (1980): 449–56.

18.   Lee and Jones, "Landfills."

19.   R. Koerner, *Designing with Geosynthetics* (Englewood Cliffs, N.J.: Prentice Hall, 1990).

20.   Joel Massmann and R. Allan Freeze, "Groundwater Contamination from Waste Management Sites: The Interaction between Risk-Based Engineering Design and Regulatory Policy. Parts 1 and 2," *Water Resources Research* 23 (1987): 351–67, 368–79.

21.   Lee and Jones, "Landfills."

22.   D. V. Lindley, *Making Decisions* (New York: Wiley-Interscience, 1971); E. A. C. Crouch and R. Wilson, *Risk/Benefit Analysis* (Cambridge, Mass.: Ballinger Publishing, 1982); R. Allan Freeze, Joel Massmann, Leslie Smith, Tony Sperling, and Bruce James, *Hydrogeological Decision Analysis* (Columbus, Ohio: National Ground Water Association, 1992).

23.   R. L. Raucher, "A Conceptual Framework for Measuring the Benefits of Groundwater Protection," *Water Resources Research* 19 (1983): 320–26.

24.   Catron et al., "Problem"; Harold A. Linstone, "On Discounting the Future," *Technological Forecasting and Social Change* 4 (1973): 335–38; R. Allan Freeze, *Groundwater Contamination: Technical Analysis and Social Decision Making*, Sixth Kisiel Lecture (University of Arizona, Department of Hydrology and Water Resources, 1987).

25.   James E. Crowfoot and Julia M. Wondolleck, *Environmental Disputes: Community Involvement in Conflict Resolution* (Washington, D.C.: Island Press, 1990).

26.   D. A. Firmage, *Modern Engineering Practice: Ethical, Professional, and Legal Aspects* (New York: Garland STPM Press, 1980), 243.

27.   Freeze, *Groundwater Contamination*.

28.   Harr, *Civil Action*.

29.   R. Gillette, "Radiation Spill at Hanford: The Anatomy of an Accident," *Science* 181 (1973): 728–30.

30.   National Academy of Sciences, *Radioactive Wastes at the Hanford Reservation: A Technical Review* (Washington, D.C.: National Academy Press, 1978).

31.   *New Yorker* (March 28, 1983).

32.   D. C. Walsh, "The History of Waste Landfilling in New York City," *Ground Water* 29 (1991): 591–93.

33.   P. E. Mariner, F. J. Holzmer, R. E. Jackson, and H. A. Meinardus, "Effects of High pH on Arsenic Mobility in a Shallow Sandy Aquifer and on Aquifer Permeability along the Adjacent Shoreline, Commencement Bay Superfund Site, Tacoma, Washington," *Environmental Science and Technology* 30 (1996): 1645–51.

34.   "U.S. Decides How to Junk Plutonium," *USA Today*, December 10, 1996.

35.   R. D. Lipschutz, *Radioactive Waste: Politics, Technology, and Risk* (Cambridge, Mass.: Ballinger Publishing, 1980).

CHAPTER 3. ENVIRONMENTAL CONTAMINATION:
WHAT MATTERS AND WHAT DOESN'T

1.   Lewis, *Technological Risk*, 126.
2.   Lehr, "Toxicological Risk"; LaGrega et al., *Hazardous Waste Management;*
Howard Holme, ed., *National Water Resources Regulation: Where Is the Environmental Pendulum Now?* (American Society of Civil Engineers, 1994); B. N. Ames,
"Six Common Errors Relating to Environmental Pollution," *Reg. Toxicol. and
Pharm.* 7 (1987): 379–80.
3.   Barnett, *Toxic Debts;* LaGrega et al., *Hazardous Waste Management;* Oakhill Environmental, *Comparison;* Office of Technology Assessment of the U.S.
Congress, *Protecting the Nation's Groundwater from Contamination,* 2 vols. (Washington, D.C.: U.S. Government Printing Office, 1984); Gabriel Britton and
Charles B. Gerba, *Groundwater Pollution Microbiology* (New York: John Wiley
and Sons, 1984); Jack E. Burbash and Elizabeth A. Resek, *Pesticides in Groundwater: Distribution, Trends, and Governing Factors* (Chelsea, Mich.: Ann Arbor
Press, 1977).
4.   W. H. Hallenback and K. M. Cunningham, *Quantitative Risk Assessment for
Environmental and Occupational Health* (Chelsea, Mich.: Lewis Publishers, 1986),
31–35.
5.   Harris, "Health Risks of Contaminated Groundwater."
6.   Lewis, *Technological Risk.*
7.   Harr, *Civil Action.*
8.   R. G. Feldman, R. M. Meyer, and A. Taub, "Evidence for Peripheral Neurotoxic Effect of Trichloroethylene," *Neurology* (June 1970); R. G. Feldman et al.,
"Long-Term Follow-Up after Single Toxic Exposure to Trichloroethylene," *Am.
Journal of Industrial Medicine* 8 (1985).
9.   Pankow and Cherry, *Dense Chlorinated Solvents,* 7–10.
10.   Lewis, *Technological Risk*, 137.
11.   "Enforcement Lax on Tap Water Purity," *San Francisco Examiner,* December
1, 1996.
12.   Office of Technology Assessment of the U.S. Congress, *Protecting the Nation's Groundwater;* P. A. Domenico and F. W. Schwartz, *Physical and Chemical
Hydrogeology,* 2d ed. (New York: Wiley, 1998), 348.
13.   Office of Technology Assessment of the U.S. Congress, *Protecting the Nation's Groundwater;* R. J. Lewis and R. L. Tatken, eds., *Registry of Toxic Effects of
Chemical Substances* (Washington, D.C.: U.S. Government Printing Office, 1980);
R. H. Harris, *The Health Risks of Toxic Organic Chemicals Found in Groundwater,*
Report No. 153 (Princeton, N.J.: Princeton University Center for Energy and En-
vironmental Studies, 1983).

14.   C. Glendenning, *When Technology Wounds* (New York: William Morrow and Company, 1990).

15.   *Science News* (July 7, 1979).

16.   Senate, Senator Larry Pressler of South Dakota, "Disposal of PCB Contaminated Liquids by the Texas Eastern Gas Pipeline Company," *Hearings of the U.S. Senate Subcommittee on Superfund and Environmental Oversight*, March 17, 1987.

17.   E. M. Whelan, *Toxic Terror: The Truth behind the Cancer Scares* (Amherst, New York: Prometheus Books, 1993), 236.

18.   Environ Corporation, *Evaluation of the Toxicology of PCBs* (Texas Eastern Toxicology Panel, 1989).

19.   Whelan, *Toxic Terror*, 237.

20.   *New York Times*, August 25, 1976.

21.   Senate, *Hearings of the U.S. Senate Subcommittee on Superfund and Environmental Oversight*.

22.   C. A. Andrews, pers. comm.

23.   Whelan, *Toxic Terror*, 242–44; D. P. Brown and M. Jones, "Mortality and Industrial Hygiene Study of Industrial Workers Exposed to Polychlorinated Biphenyls," *Archives of Environmental Health* 36 (1981): 120.

24.   U.S. Public Health Service, *ToxFAQs: Polychlorinated Biphenyls* (Washington, D.C.: Government Printing Office, 1993).

25.   P. H. Abelson, "Excessive Fear of PCBs," *Science* 253 (1991): 361.

26.   Frank Wania and Donald Mackay, "Tracking the Distribution of Persistent Organic Pollutants," *Environmental Science and Technology News* 30 (1996): 390–96A.

27.   Theo Colborn, Diane Dumanoski, and John Peterson Myers, *Our Stolen Future* (New York: Dutton, 1996).

28.   Whelan, *Toxic Terror*, 244–45.

29.   Jane E. Brody, "Report Links PCB Exposure with Children's Development," *New York Times*, September 12, 1996.

30.   Pankow and Cherry, *Dense Chlorinated Solvents*, 14.

31.   Lehr, "Toxicological Risk."

32.   LaGrega et al., *Hazardous Waste Management*, 247.

33.   Hallenback and Cunningham, *Quantitative Risk Assessment*.

34.   Ibid., 46.

35.   LaGrega et al., *Hazardous Waste Management*, 61.

36.   *Wall Street Journal*, February 24, 1995; Howard Holme, "Risk Assessment and Cost-Benefit Analysis Are Keys to Environmental Law Reform" (paper presented at the American Society of Civil Engineers 22nd Annual Conference, Cambridge, Mass., May 9, 1995).

37.   C. W. Fetter, *Contaminant Hydrogeology* (Englewood Cliffs, N.J.: Prentice Hall, 1993).

38.   Lehr, "Toxicological Risk"; Holme, "Risk Assessment"; Dennis J. Pausten-

bach, "Health Risk Assessments: Opportunities and Pitfalls," *Columbia Journal of Environmental Law* 14 (1989): 379–410.

39. Holme, "Risk Assessment."

40. Lewis, *Technological Risk,* 79.

41. Ibid.

42. Lehr, "Toxicological Risk."

43. Harris, "Health Risks of Contaminated Groundwater."

44. Hallenback and Cunningham, *Quantitative Risk Assessment;* U.S. Environmental Protection Agency, *Risk Assessment Guidance for Superfund, Volume 1: Human Health Evaluation Manual, Part A,* EPA/540/1–89/002 (Washington, D.C.: U.S. Government Printing Office, 1989).

45. Ibid.

46. Holme, "Risk Assessment."

47. Ibid.

48. Donald A. Brown, "The Urgent Need to Integrate Ethical Considerations into Risk Assessment Procedures," in *Handbook for Environmental Risk Decision Making: Values, Perceptions, and Ethics,* ed. C. Richard Cothern (Boca Raton: CRC Press, 1996), 115–25.

49. C. Richard Cothern, "An Overview of Environmental Risk Decision Making: Values, Perceptions, and Ethics," in *Handbook for Environmental Risk Decision Making: Values, Perceptions, and Ethics,* ed. C. Richard Cothern (Boca Raton: CRC Press, 1996).

50. Lester B. Lave, "Economic Tools for Risk Reduction," in *Societal Risk Assessment: How Safe Is Safe Enough?* ed. Richard C. Schwing and Walter A. Albers Jr. (New York: Plenum Press, 1980), 115–28.

51. Lehr, "Toxicological Risk."

52. Robert S. Raucher, "The Economic Value of Groundwater Protection: What Are the Benefits and How Do They Compare to the Costs?" *GSA Today* 3 (July 1993): 183–94.

53. Paul Slovic, Baruch Fischoff, and Sarah Lichtenstein, "Facts and Fears: Understanding Perceived Risk," in *Societal Risk Assessment: How Safe Is Safe Enough?* ed. Richard C. Schwing and Walter A. Albers Jr. (New York: Plenum Press, 1980), 181–211.

54. Bruce N. Ames, Renae Magaw, and Lois Swirsky Gold, "Ranking Possible Carcinogenic Hazards," *Science* 236 (1987): 271–76.

55. Harris, "Health Risks of Contaminated Groundwater"; Fetter, *Contaminant;* Richard Wilson, "Analyzing the Daily Risks of Life," *Technology Review* (February 1979).

56. Lehr, "Toxicological Risk"; Wilson, "Analyzing the Daily Risks."

57. Cothern, "Overview"; Slovic, Fischoff, and Lichtenstein, "Facts."

58. LaGrega et al., *Hazardous Waste Management,* 865.

59. Slovic, Fischoff, and Lichtenstein, "Facts."

60.   *Vancouver Sun,* May 29, 1980.

61.   Lewis, *Technological Risk,* 79.

62.   B. Fischoff, S. Lichtenstein, P. Slovic, S. L. Derby, and R. L. Keeney, *Acceptable Risk* (New York: Cambridge University Press, 1981).

63.   David J. Cushman and Stephen D. Ball, "Groundwater Modeling for Risk-Assessment Purposes," *Ground Water Monitoring and Remediation* 13, no. 4 (1993): 162–72.

64.   Shrader-Frechette, *Risk.*

65.   E. F. Schumacher, *Small Is Beautiful* (New York: Harper and Row, 1973), 46.

66.   Fischoff et al., *Acceptable Risk;* Freeze, *Groundwater Contamination;* Mark Sharefkin, Mordechai Schecter, and Allen Kneese, "Impacts, Costs, and Techniques for Mitigation of Contaminated Groundwater: A Review," *Water Resources Research* 20 (1984): 1771–83.

67.   Sharefkin et al., "Impacts."

68.   Catron et al., "Problem."

69.   Aaron Wildavsky, *Searching for Safety* (New Brunswick, NJ: Transaction Publishers, 1988).

70.   John F. Morrall III, "A Review of the Record," *Regulation* (November-December 1986), as quoted in Holme, "Risk Assessment."

71.   Holme, "Risk Assessment."

72.   Sharefkin et al., "Impacts"; Richard C. Schwing, "Trade-Offs," in *Societal Risk Assessment: How Safe Is Safe Enough?* ed. Richard C. Schwing and Walter A. Albers Jr. (New York: Plenum Press, 1980), 129–41.

73.   T. O. Tengs et al., *Five Hundred Life-Saving Interventions and Their Cost Effectiveness* (Harvard Center for Risk Analysis, 1994).

74.   Schwing, "Trade-Offs."

75.   Hird, *Superfund,* 95.

76.   Ibid.

77.   Raucher, "Economic Value."

78.   U.S. Environmental Protection Agency, *Unfinished Business: A Comparative Assessment of Environmental Problems* (Washington, D.C.: U.S. Government Printing Office, February 1987).

79.   U.S. Environmental Protection Agency, Science Advisory Board, *Reducing Risk: Setting Priorities and Strategies for Environmental Protection* (Washington, D.C.: U.S. Government Printing Office, September 1990).

80.   "New Air Quality Standards Generate Heat," *EOS, Transactions of the American Geophysical Union* 78 (April 15, 1997): 153.

81.   LaGrega et al., *Hazardous Waste Management.*

82.   Lehr, "Toxicological Risk."

CHAPTER 4. THE UNPLEASANT TRUTHS ABOUT WASTE MANAGEMENT

1. J. F. Pankow, Stan Feenstra, John A. Cherry, and M. Cathryn Ryan, "Dense Chlorinated Solvents in Groundwater: Background and History of the Problem," in *Dense Chlorinated Solvents and Other DNAPLs in Groundwater: History, Behavior, and Remediation,* ed. James F. Pankow and John A. Cherry (Waterloo, Ont.: Waterloo Press, 1996).

2. Ibid.

3. Ibid.

4. Ibid.

5. Harr, *Civil Action.*

6. Barnett, *Toxic Debts,* 23–28; LaGrega et al., *Hazardous Waste Management,* 22–24.

7. John A. Cherry, "Who Is to Blame and What Can Be Done?" *GSA Today* 3 (September 1993): 233–34.

8. Charles A. Job, "Benefits and Costs of Wellhead Protection," *Ground Water Monitoring and Remediation* 16 (spring 1996): 65–68; U.S. Environmental Protection Agency, *Benefits and Costs of Prevention: Case Studies of Community Wellhead Protection,* EPA Report No. 813-B-95–005 (Washington, D.C.: U.S. Government Printing Office, 1995).

9. Barnett, *Toxic Debts,* 92–94.

10. Office of Technology Assessment of the U.S. Congress, *Groundwater Protection Standards for Hazardous Waste Land Disposal Facilities: Will They Prevent More Superfund Sites?* (Office of Technology Assessment of the U.S. Congress, staff memorandum, April 6, 1984).

11. Linda E. Greer, "Groundwater Pollution Prevention: Putting Our Money Where Our Mouth Is," *GSA Today* 3 (July 1993): 179–81.

12. Job, "Benefits"; W. J. McCabe, C. A. Job, J. J. Simons, J. S. Graves, and C. J. Terada, "History of the Sole Source Aquifer Program: A Community-Based Approach for Protecting Aquifers Used for Drinking Water Supply," *Ground Water Monitoring and Remediation* 17 (summer 1997): 78–86.

13. Rathje and Murphy, *Rubbish!* 197.

14. Brown, *Laying Waste,* 272.

15. Rathje and Murphy, *Rubbish!* 211.

16. Ibid., 239.

17. LaGrega et al., *Hazardous Waste Management;* Moni Campbell, "Industrial Waste Reduction and Recovery," *Alternatives* 10 (1982): 59–64; Lawrence Smith and Jeffrey Means, *Recycling and Reuse of Industrial Waste* (Columbus, Ohio: Battelle Press, 1995).

18.   Campbell, ibid.

19.   Ibid.

20.   Ibid.

21.   Rathje and Murphy, *Rubbish!* 210.

22.   Brown, *Laying Waste*, 273.

23.   Rathje and Murphy, *Rubbish!* 85.

24.   Lee and Jones, "Landfills."

25.   D. R. Burman, P. V. Roberts, and D. M. Mackay, *Estimating the Impact of Policy Decisions on Hazardous Waste Landfill Performance* (Stanford: Department of Civil Engineering, Stanford University, 1985).

26.   Oakhill Environmental, *Comparison;* D. C. Wilson, *Waste Management: Planning, Evaluation, Technologies* (Oxford University Press, 1981); G. Farquhar, F. Rovers, and E. McBean, *Solid Waste Landfill Engineering and Design* (Englewood Cliffs, N.J.: Prentice Hall, 1996).

27.   Oakhill Environmental, *Comparison.*

28.   Wilson, *Waste,* 199.

29.   Domenico and Schwartz, *Physical and Chemical Hydrogeology;* Pankow and Cherry, *Dense Chlorinated Solvents;* Fetter, *Contaminant;* R. A. Freeze and J. A. Cherry, *Groundwater* (Englewood Cliffs, N.J.: Prentice Hall, 1979); S. C. Hern and S. M. Melancon, *Vadose-Zone Modeling of Organic Pollutants* (Chelsea, Mich.: Lewis Publishers, 1986); L. J. Thibodeaux, *Chemodynamics: Environmental Movement of Chemicals in Air, Water, and Soil* (New York: Wiley, 1979).

30.   Pankow and Cherry, *Dense Chlorinated Solvents;* Domenico and Schwartz, *Physical and Chemical Hydrogeology;* Fetter, *Contaminant;* J. W. Mercer and R. M. Cohen, "A Review of Immiscible Fluids in the Subsurface: Properties, Models, Characterization, and Remediation," *Journal of Contaminant Hydrology* 6 (1990): 107–63.

31.   Pankow and Cherry, *Dense Chlorinated Solvents,* 480.

32.   Freeze and Cherry, *Groundwater.*

33.   D. R. LeBlanc, ed., *Movement and Fate of Solutes in a Plume of Sewage-Contaminated Groundwater, Cape Cod, Massachusetts,* U.S. Geological Survey Open File Report 84–475 (Washington, D.C.: U.S. Government Printing Office, 1984).

34.   J. A. Cherry, ed., "Migration of Contaminants in Groundwater at a Landfill: A Case Study," *Journal of Hydrology* 63, nos. 1-2 (1983).

35.   Massmann and Freeze, "Groundwater."

36.   Lee and Jones, "Landfills."

37.   J. H. Lehr, "South Dakota Is the Answer. What Is the Question?" *Ground Water* 29 (1991): 322–26.

38.   Rathje and Murphy, *Rubbish!* 109.

39.   Garrett Hardin, "The Tragedy of the Commons," *Science* 162 (December 13, 1968).

40.   Rathje and Murphy, *Rubbish!* 107.

41.   Mazmanian and Morell, *Beyond Superfailure,* 180.

42.   Walsh, "History."

43.   Elizabeth Royte, "Other People's Garbage: The New Politics of Trash: A Case Study," *Harper's Magazine* (June 1992): 54–60.

44.   Larry W. Cantor and Robert C. Knox, *Ground Water Pollution Control* (Chelsea, Mich.: Lewis Publishers, 1986); M. L. O'Hare, L. Bacon, and D. Sanderson, *Facility Siting and Public Opposition* (New York: Van Nostrand Rheinhold, 1983); D. A. Walker, *An Approach to the Management of Groundwater Pollution* (Ph.D. diss., University of British Columbia, 1996).

45.   R. N. L. Andrews, "Hazardous Waste Facility Siting: State Approaches," in *Dimensions of Hazardous Waste Politics and Policy,* ed. Charles E. Davis and James P. Lester (Westport, Conn.: Greenwood Press, 1988).

46.   Ibid.; Mazmanian and Morell, *Beyond Superfailure,* 186–91.

47.   C. B. Andersen and B. Polkinghorn, "Geology as a Social Science: Addressing the Complexity of Human Habits and Values in Water Quality Conflicts," *GSA Today* 6 (April 1996): 36–38.

48.   K. E. Portney, "The Role of Economic Factors in Lay Perceptions of Risk," in *Dimensions of Hazardous Waste Politics and Policy,* ed. Charles E. Davis and James P. Lester (Westport, Conn.: Greenwood Press, 1988).

49.   Chris Zeiss and James Atwater, "Waste Facilities in Residential Communities: Impacts and Acceptance," *American Society of Civil Engineers Journal of Urban Planning and Development* 113 (1987): 19–34.

50.   Barry G. Rabe, *Beyond NIMBY: Hazardous Waste Siting in Canada and the United States* (Washington, D.C.: Brookings Institution, 1994), 61–89.

51.   Mazmanian and Morell, *Beyond Superfailure,* 191.

52.   Lester Thurow, *The Zero-Sum Society* (New York: Basic Books, 1980).

53.   Royte, "Other People's Garbage."

54.   Colin Crawford, *Uproar at Dancing Rabbit Creek: Battling over Race, Class, and the Environment* (Reading, Mass.: Addison Wesley, 1996).

55.   John B. Robertson and Howard Wilshire, "Is Ward Valley Safe? A Point/Counterpoint Discussion," *Geotimes* (June 1997): 18–23.

56.   National Research Council, *Rethinking High-Level Radioactive Waste Disposal* (Washington, D.C.: National Academy Press, 1990).

57.   James Flynn, Roger Kasperson, Howard Kunreuther, and Paul Slovic, "Time to Rethink Nuclear Waste Storage," *Issues in Science and Technology* (summer 1992): 42–48.

58.   Ibid.; National Research Council, *Rethinking High-Level Radioactive;* R. D. Lipschutz, *Radioactive Waste: Politics, Technology and Risk* (Cambridge, Mass.: Ballinger Publishing, 1980); K. F. Weaver, "The Promise and Peril of Nuclear Energy," *National Geographic* 155 (1979): 459–93.

59.   Ford Foundation, *Nuclear Power.*

60.   National Academy of Sciences Committee on Waste Disposal, *The Disposal of Radioactive Waste on Land,* National Research Council Publ. 519 (Washington, D.C.: National Academy Press, 1957).

61.   Flynn et al., "Time."

62.   Lipschutz, *Radioactive Waste.*

63.   Medvedev, *Legacy.*

64.   U.S. Department of Energy, *Repository Safety Strategy: U.S. Department of Energy's Strategy to Protect Public Health and Safety after Closure of a Yucca Mountain Repository,* Report YMP/96–01 (Washington, D.C.: U.S. Government Printing Office, 1998).

65.   J. W. Mercer, S. D. Thomas, and B. Ross, *Parameters and Variables Appearing in Repository Siting Models,* U.S. Nuclear Regulatory Commission, NUREG/CR-3066 (Washington, D.C.: U.S. Government Printing Office, 1982).

66.   Sandia National Laboratories, *Total-System Performance Analysis for Yucca Mountain,* Report SAND93–2675 (Albuquerque, N.M.: Sandia National Laboratories, 1994).

67.   G. I. Rochlin, "Nuclear Waste Disposal: Two Social Criteria," *Science* 195 (1977): 23–31.

68.   U.S. Department of Energy, *Repository.*

69.   Flynn et al., "Time."

70.   National Academy of Sciences, *The Waste Isolation Pilot Plant: A Potential Solution for the Disposal of Transuranic Waste,* National Research Council (Washington, D.C.: National Academy Press, 1996).

71.   K. W. Dormuth, P. A. Gillespie, and S. H. Whitaker, "Disposal of Nuclear Fuel Waste," *Issues in Environmental Science and Technology,* no. 3 (1995): 115–30.

72.   Lewis, *Technological Risk,* 247.

73.   E. W. Colglazier, ed., *The Politics of Nuclear Waste* (New York: Pergamon Press, 1982); L. Carter, *Nuclear Imperatives and Public Trust: Dealing with Radioactive Waste* (Washington, D.C.: Resources for the Future, 1987); G. Jacob, *Site Unseen: The Politics of Siting a Nuclear Waste Repository* (Pittsburgh: University of Pittsburgh Press, 1990).

CHAPTER 5.   THE UNPLEASANT TRUTHS
ABOUT REMEDIATION

1.   Cherry, "Who Is to Blame."

2.   Sharefkin, Schecter, and Kneese, "Impacts."

3.   Ibid.

4.   J. W. Mercer, David C. Skipp, and Daniel Giffen, *Basics of Pump-and-Treat*

Ground-Water Remediation Technology, U.S. Environmental Protection Agency, EPA-600/8–90/003 (Washington, D.C.: U.S. Government Printing Office, 1990).

5.   Ibid.

6.   J. A. Cherry, S. Feenstra, and D. M. Mackay, "Developing Rational Goals for In-Situ Remedial Technologies," in *Subsurface Restoration,* ed. C. H. Ward, J. A. Cherry, and M. R. Scalf (Chelsea, Mich.: Ann Arbor Press, 1997).

7.   Pankow and Cherry, *Dense Chlorinated Solvents;* R. A. Freeze and D. B. McWhorter, "A Framework for Assessing Risk Reduction Due to DNAPL Mass Removal from Low-Permeability Soils," *Ground Water* 35 (1997): 111–23.

8.   Pankow and Cherry, *Dense Chlorinated Solvents,* 475–505; C. H. Ward, J. A. Cherry, and M. R. Scalf, eds., *Subsurface Restoration* (Chelsea, Mich.: Ann Arbor Press, 1997); G. Grubb and N. Sitar, *Evaluation of Technologies for In-Situ Cleanup of DNAPL Contaminated Sites,* U.S. Environmental Protection Agency, EPA/600/ R-94/120 (Washington, D.C.: U.S. Government Printing Office, 1994); Stephen M. Testa and Duane L. Winegardner, *Restoration of Petroleum Contaminated Aquifers* (Chelsea, Mich.: Lewis Publishers, 1991); National Research Council, *Innovations in Groundwater and Soil Cleanup: From Concept to Commercialization* (Washington, D.C.: National Academy Press, 1997); J. A. MacDonald and P. S. Rao, "Shift Needed to Improve Market for Innovative Technologies," *Soil and Groundwater Cleanup* (August-September 1997): 19–25.

9.   K. S. Udell, "Thermally Enhanced Removal of Liquid Hydrocarbon," in *Subsurface Restoration,* ed. C. H. Ward, J. A. Cherry, and M. R. Scalf (Chelsea, Mich.: Ann Arbor Press, 1997), 251–70; Grubb and Sitar, *Evaluation.*

10.   J. C. Fountain, "Removal of Nonaqueous Phase Liquids Using Surfactants," in *Subsurface Restoration,* ed. C. H. Ward, J. A. Cherry, and M. R. Scalf (Chelsea, Mich.: Ann Arbor Press, 1997), 199–207.

11.   D. C. M. Augustijn, L. S. Lee, R. E. Jessup, P. S. C. Rao, M. D. Annable, and A. L. Wood, "Remediation of Soils and Aquifers Contaminated with Organic Chemicals: Theoretical Basis for the Use of Cosolvents," in *Subsurface Restoration,* ed. C. H. Ward, J. A. Cherry, and M. R. Scalf (Chelsea, Mich.: Ann Arbor Press, 1997), 231–50.

12.   Robert E. Hinchee, ed., *Air Sparging for Site Restoration* (Columbus, Ohio: Battelle Press, 1993); R. A. Brown, "Air Sparging: A Primer for Application and Design," in *Subsurface Restoration,* ed. C. H. Ward, J. A. Cherry and M. R. Scalf (Chelsea, Mich.: Ann Arbor Press, 1997), 301–27.

13.   Udell, "Thermally Enhanced Removal."

14.   Fountain, "Removal."

15.   Grubb and Sitar, *Evaluation.*

16.   J. Becker, "Throwing a Blanket on the Problem," *Soil and Groundwater Cleanup* (May 1997): 6–11.

17.   Pankow and Cherry, *Dense Chlorinated Solvents,* 501.

18.   Ibid.; A. R. Gavaskar, *Permeable Barriers for Groundwater Remediation* (Columbus, Ohio: Battelle Press, 1997); R. W. Gillham and D. R. Burris, "Recent Developments in Permeable In-Situ Treatment Walls for Remediation of Contaminated Groundwater," in *Subsurface Restoration*, ed. C. H. Ward, J. A. Cherry, and M. R. Scalf (Chelsea, Mich.: Ann Arbor Press, 1997), 343–56.

19.   R. W. Gillham and S. F. O'Hannesin, "Enhanced Degradation of Halogenated Aliphatics by Zero-Valent Iron," *Ground Water* 32 (1994): 958–67.

20.   National Research Council, *In Situ Bioremediation: When Does It Work?* (Washington, D.C.: National Academy Press, 1993).

21.   Union Pacific Railroad, *In Situ Treatment Process Development Program, Laramie Tie Plant, Milestone IV Report* (N.p., Union Pacific Railroad, August 1990).

22.   U.S. Environmental Protection Agency, *Guidance for Evaluating the Technical Impracticability of Groundwater Restoration*, Interim Final OSWER Directive 9234.2–25 (Washington, D.C.: U.S. Government Printing Office, 1993).

23.   Jan Kay, "Bay Area's Worst Pollution," *San Francisco Examiner*, December 1, 1996.

24.   *San Luis Obispo New Times*, November 7, 1996.

25.   J. A. Cherry, S. Feenstra, and D. M. Mackay, "Concepts for the Remediation of Sites Contaminated with DNAPLs," in *Dense Chlorinated Solvents and Other DNAPLs in Groundwater* (Waterloo, Ont.: Waterloo Press, 1996), pp. 475–506.

CHAPTER 6.
THE REGULATORY QUAGMIRE

1.   Philip K. Howard, *Death of Common Sense: How Law Is Suffocating America* (New York: Warner Books, 1994), 47.

2.   Thurow, *Zero-Sum Society*.

3.   Ibid.

4.   Robert L. Raucher, "A Conceptual Framework for Measuring the Benefits of Groundwater Protection," *Water Resources Research* 19 (1983): 320–26.

5.   Shrader-Frechette, *Risk*, 131–45.

6.   Howard, *Death of Common Sense*, 22.

7.   Holme, "Risk Assessment."

8.   Volokh and Marzulla, *Environmental Enforcement*.

9.   Walsh, "History."

10.   W. Duvel, "The Brownfields Initiative," *Soil and Groundwater Cleanup* (August-September 1997): 9–10.

11.   Timothy M. O'Connor and Gregory S. Fine, "Brownfields Program Works to State's Benefit in Rhode Island," *Soil and Groundwater Cleanup* (August-September 1997), 32–44.

12. *Air and Water Pollution Report* (newsletter), July 25, 1994.

13. Marianne Lavelle, "Environmental Vise: Law, Compliance," *National Law Journal* (August 30, 1993): 88.

14. LaGrega et al., *Hazardous Waste Management*, 41.

15. Office of Technology Assessment of the U.S. Congress, *Groundwater*.

16. Hird, *Superfund*, 22–23.

17. R. Allan Freeze and John A. Cherry, "What Has Gone Wrong?" *Ground Water* 27 (1989): 458–64; R. A. Hodge and A. J. Roman, "Ground-Water Protection Policies: Myths and Alternatives," *Ground Water* 28 (1990): 498–504.

18. Howard, *Death of Common Sense*, 179.

19. Dieter, *Engineering Design*.

20. Hird, *Superfund*, 10.

21. Mazmanian and Morell, *Beyond Superfailure*, 7; Hird, *Superfund*, 27.

22. LaGrega et al., *Hazardous Waste Management*, 55; Hird, *Superfund*, 29.

23. Hird, *Superfund*, 29.

24. James R. Janis and Edwin Berk, "Superfund: Significant Accomplishments," *Ground Water* 25 (1987): 2–11.

25. Freeze and Cherry, "What Has Gone Wrong?"

26. Mazmanian and Morell, *Beyond Superfailure*.

27. Thomas W. Church and Robert T. Nakamura, *Cleaning Up the Mess: Implementation Strategies in Superfund* (Washington, D.C.: Brookings Institution, 1993), 164.

28. Ibid., 38.

29. P. E. Mariner, F. J. Holzmer, R. E. Jackson, H. W. Meinardus, and F. W. Wolf, "Effects of High pH on Arsenic Mobility in a Shallow Sandy Aquifer and on Aquifer Permeability along the Adjacent Shoreline, Commencement Bay Superfund Site, Tacoma, Washington," *Environmental Science and Technology* 30 (1996): 1645–51.

30. J. L. Sadd, T. Boer, M. Pastor Jr., and L. D. Snyder, "Assessing Environmental Justice: The Demographics of Hazardous Waste in Los Angeles County," *GSA Today* 7 (August 1997): 18–19.

31. Hird, *Superfund*, 190.

32. Ibid.; Joel S. Hirschhorn, "Superfund: A Scientifically Sound Strategy Needed," *Ground Water* 25 (1987): 3–11.

33. Hird, *Superfund*, 212.

34. Job, "Benefits"; John R. Odermatt, "Back to Basics in Environmental Protection," *Ground Water* 33 (1995): 354–55; John R. Odermatt, "Effective Implementation of the Watershed Management Approach for Adjudicated Ground Water Basins in California," *Ground Water Monitoring and Remediation* 17 (spring 1997): 73–76.

35. "Enforcement Lax on Tap Water Purity," *San Francisco Examiner*, December 2, 1996.

36.   U.S. Environmental Protection Agency, *Unfinished Business*; U.S. Environmental Protection Agency, *Reducing Risk*.
37.   Hird, *Superfund*, 8.
38.   Jocelyn White, "Superfund: Pouring Money Down a Hole," *New York Times*, April 17, 1992.

CHAPTER 7.   THE ENVIRONMENTAL GAME

1.   Hird, *Superfund*.
2.   "Cleaning Up," *Atlantic* 266, no. 4 (1990): 46–50.
3.   Walker, "Approach."
4.   Marcel Moreau, "A Regulator's Perspective on Prevention of Leaks from Underground Storage Systems, Maine Department of Environmental Protection" (manuscript, 1985).
5.   Walker, "Approach."
6.   J. H. Frost and W. W. Wilmot, *Interpersonal Conflict* (Dubuque, Iowa: William C. Brown Company Publishers, 1978); P. Wehr, *Conflict Regulation* (Boulder, Colo.: Westview Press, 1979).
7.   Walker, "Approach"; R. Fisher, W. Ury, and B. Patton, *Getting to Yes* (New York: Penguin Books, 1991); H. Raiffa, *The Art and Science of Negotiation* (Cambridge: Harvard University Press, 1982); L. Susskind and J. Cruikshank, *Breaking the Impasse: Consensual Approaches to Resolving Public Disputes* (New York: Basic Books, 1987); J. L. Creighton and J. Delli Priscoli, eds., *Public Involvement Techniques: A Reader of Ten Years' Experience at the Institute of Water Resources*, U.S. Army Institute for Water Resources, IWR Staff Report 81–1, 1981.
8.   C. W. Wolfram, *Modern Legal Ethics* (St. Paul, Minn.: West Publishing, 1982).
9.   Howard, *Death of Common Sense*, 86.
10.   *USA Today*, November 6, 1996.
11.   Firmage, *Modern Engineering*, 246.
12.   Peter W. Huber, *Galileo's Revenge: Junk Science in the Courtroom* (New York: Basic Books, 1991), 19.
13.   Ibid.
14.   Ibid., 18.
15.   Ibid.
16.   Francisco J. Ayala and Bert Black, "Science and the Courts," *American Scientist* 81 (1993): 230–39; Peter J. Neufeld and Neville Coleman, "When Science Takes the Witness Stand," *Scientific American* 262 (1990): 46–53.
17.   Ayala and Black, "Science."

18.   Thurow, *Zero-Sum Society*, 13.

19.   MacDonald and Rao, "Shift."

20.   Firmage, *Modern Engineering*, 243.

21.   Warren W. Wood, "A Question of Ethics," *Ground Water* 34 (1996): 385; R. E. Jackson, "Comments on 'A Question of Ethics' by Warren W. Wood," *Ground Water* 35 (1997): 4–5.

22.   *British Columbia Professional Engineer* (December 1996).

23.   Rathje and Murphy, *Rubbish!* 85.

24.   Brown, *Laying Waste*, 248.

25.   Ibid.

26.   Mazmanian and Morell, *Beyond Superfailure*.

27.   T. W. Rothermal, "Pitfalls in the Hazardous Waste Management Business," *Environmental Progress* 2 (1983): 221–25.

28.   Center for Investigative Reporting and Bill Moyers, *Global Dumping Ground: The International Traffic in Hazardous Waste* (Washington: Seven Locks Press, 1990).

29.   "Smuggling of Banned Chemical Threatens Ozone," *Vancouver Sun*, January 10, 1997.

30.   Volokh and Marzulla, *Environmental Enforcement*.

Index

Text: Palatino
Display: Bauer Bodoni and Snell Roundhand Script
Composition: Binghamton Valley Composition
Printing and binding: BookCrafters
Figures: Bill Nelson